SH
BEYOND
CANCER

7 STEPS TO LIVING A BETTER LIFE

LISA DIMOND AND MARC SLUGH

Shine Beyond Cancer
The 7 Secrets to Living Your Best Life
Lisa Dimond and Marc Slugh

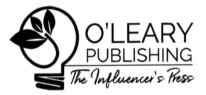

For bulk group pricing please email: info@shinebeyondcancer.com

This book is not intended as a substitute for the medical advice of physicians. The reader should regularly consult a physician in matters relating to his/her health and particularly with respect to any symptoms that may require diagnosis or medical attention.

The views, information, or opinions expressed in this book are solely those of the authors involved and do not necessarily represent those of O'Leary Publishing, LLC.

ISBN: 978-1-68454-115-7

Cover Design by Christine Dupre
Photography by Julie Renner
Interior Design by Lisa Thomson
Editing by Dalton Fisher
Copy Editing by Joy Xiang

Printed in the United States of America

Dedicated to You

May Shine Beyond Cancer spark the hope and inspiration
you need to live your best life, full of health, love, and joy.

This is our intention for you.

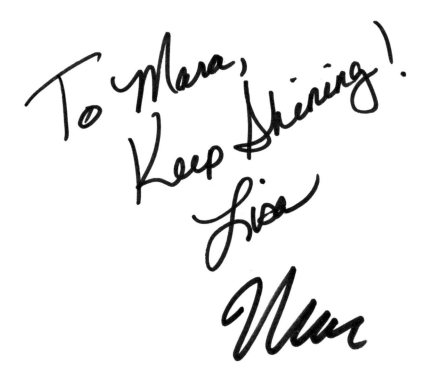

To Mara,
Keep Shining!.
Lisa

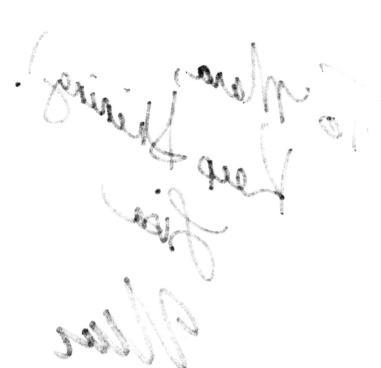

TABLE OF CONTENTS

FOREWORD

Going through cancer is not easy. And it's not easy for those you love either. This foreword was written as a complete surprise to Marc and Lisa. In fact, they didn't even see it until the interior came back from the designer for them to review one last time. Yes, we were that sneaky!

They deserve every word written and every bit of love and appreciation that appears on the following pages. Special thank you to Danielle Russo-Slugh, Marc's wife, for collecting all the love letters. With no further ado, we introduce you to those who know the authors best...starting with a letter from Danielle and then Lisa's two daughters and finally Marc's five children. Enjoy.

April O'Leary
O'Leary Publishing

Dear Marc,

As we approach our 20 year anniversary in a few short months, it's amazing to see this labor of love come into the world. I have loved the journey of life with you. Just like the wedding vows say *through sickness and health, for rich or for poor*, we've tested all combinations and still managed to come out on top. More in love, more connected, able to navigate uncertainty, and choose to live a life in contribution. You have been open to growing together which has been the only way we could have survived this long journey with the challenges we've faced. You have taught me it's ok to choose what fulfills you and not chase what doesn't.

You have been the inspiration for our family to SHINE and THRIVE. When you partnered with Lisa I could see a whole new spark in you as you threw yourself into this much-needed work. You both have authentically put your heart and soul into this for one reason only, to pay it forward and help others SHINE powerfully. You are two of the most giving, loving, compassionate people I know. My wish is that this project will touch so many lives and lift people up through your inspiration, energy, and example. *I am as always your biggest fan, supporter, and cheerleader.*

I love you and I am so proud of you!

xo Danielle

To Our Beautiful Momma,

We can't believe we are here five years later, five years cancer-free. It has been one incredible journey filled with tears, laughs and a whole lotta wine. You inspired us with every step you took and every stride you made. Not only did you inspire us, but you also taught us what it means to be strong, caring individuals even when nothing was going our way. You made it look so easy, but we know it was not. We truly did not know what strength looked like until we had a front-row seat to this journey.

You are our cheerleader, coach, therapist, home cook, nurse, and biggest supporter. How scary to lose all of that in one's life. But we didn't and for that, we are forever grateful. Your positivity was your most successful medicine, and many people can learn from that.

Thank you for making us stronger women and showing us what it means to be better sisters, daughters, and friends. We can't wait to see you continue to shine your light beyond cancer and help many more along the way.

We love you more than you'll ever know, and there will never be enough ways to show that. Thank you for all of the love that you have and continue to give us every day. We are the luckiest girls in the world and hope to be half the woman that you are someday.

Love you always,
Veronica & Olivia

Dear Dad,

Growing up, I always thought that nothing could or would ever happen to you. To be honest, I still feel that way. I cannot imagine living one day without being able to call or text you to vent about my day or to get level-headed advice.

In August 2006, right before I left for my first year of college, you had a heart attack. I was scared and most of all disappointed that you couldn't bring me to Arizona for college, and this is when I started to realize that you weren't as invincible as I thought. I thought about all the awful things that could happen as a result of that heart attack, especially while I was away at college. But you proved to be invincible and came out of that heart attack like the hero that you are. And then double-proved yourself by coming to Arizona to kick butt in a beer pong tournament with my college freshman friends!

Five years later, on the day before my second year of teaching, you scared me again. When you called to tell me that you had cancer, stage 4 cancer to be exact, I fell apart. Thoughts of death and hospitals came to my mind, and all you said was, "Enough about me, tell me about your classroom and what you're doing on the first day of school." And that is how your attitude remained throughout your fight against cancer. You have shown me through your kindness, selfless acts, and an outpouring of love that life can be unpredictable.

I am so proud to brag about you and your fight against cancer because I know how badly you want to help others.

Thank you for not letting anything happen to you and proving your invincibility, because there is no one else who gives me rational advice like you.

I love you!
Love always,
Sam

Dear Dad,

When asked to write a letter about how I felt during your cancer diagnosis, I immediately froze. It is very hard to put into words how I felt. However, two words come to mind, and all I have to say is…THANK YOU.

THANK YOU for showing me true strength.

THANK YOU for showing me that there is no option to give up.

THANK YOU for always having a positive attitude through it all.

THANK YOU for looking handsome even when you're bald with no eyebrows.

THANK YOU for being so generous and selfless.

Dad, you are the strongest man I know, and you have proved to me that you can overcome anything life throws your way. I am eternally grateful for you and beyond thankful that you chose me to be your daughter.

F**K cancer, man.

I LOVE YOU!

Love,
DJ

Dear Daddy,

I have been sitting here for a few minutes now, trying to figure out how I can even put into words how much I admire you. I kept typing, hitting the backspace and then typing again. I think it was so difficult for me to start this letter to you because I have so many thoughts to share that I did not know where to start!

I admire you for your bravery. Going through cancer must have been so terrifying and scary. You did not make it seem that way. You continued to put a smile on your face, despite the fear you were feeling.

I admire your positivity. You have five kids, a wife, a house, a dog and you still manage to remain positive through it all. You are always my go-to when I need encouragement and motivation.

I admire your generosity. You are always going above and beyond when it comes to giving back or helping others in need. That is a trait that I find the most admirable about you.

I am the luckiest girl to have a dad like you to look up to every day. I love you to the moon.

Love,
Your Original Baby (Brittles)

Dear Dad,

I don't know if you remember this, but this story made me realize that this treatment was not a joke.

One day on a beautiful morning on Long Beach Island in the summer, I was playing with my hockey action figures, ready to go to the beach. You walked into my room to check on me. As you called my name, I turned around and looked at you. You were shivering, your skin was pale and you were wearing a winter coat. It was ninety degrees out and I asked you, "Dad, why are you shivering?" You said, "I don't know." This was when I figured out why you were in the hospital and why mom was so worried.

Rewind a little bit. I remember the day that mom told Sarah and me about this "special sickness" that you had received two weeks prior. At that point, I was young and I didn't really know what it was or what the effects and outcomes could be. When you had to undergo the process of healing, we visited you in the hospital in NYC every weekend and waited to hear what the weekly report from the doctor was. I remember all I cared about was when you would get out of the hospital and back home to be my hockey goalie. On the way home from the hospital, Sarah and I would ask mom questions about you and try to understand why you were there for so long.

Fast forward about a year and a half later, I remember the day I was getting ready for practice and you got off the phone and told Sarah, mom and me that you would have to go through the fourth chemo treatment, and how your health was getting much better. With this treatment, you would have significant chances to kick cancer out of your body. About seven weeks later, I walked into that hospital. Mom was the happiest she had been in two years! She didn't tell Sarah and me what was happening; she just urged us to see you. You were cancer-free! I walked out of that building in NYC and I never saw that hospital again. Mom cried tears that you were finally in good condition as we went through the Holland Tunnel. Sarah and I celebrated because we would get to see you and play with you every single day now. We were back to being a happy family.

Around two years later, I finally understood what happened to you and I understood more about the actual disease itself in school. I learned about the potential outcomes of what could have happened. It was then that I thought, *what if I didn't have a person to tie my skates or be my goalie when I wanted to practice my moves?*

Today when I walk around the house, I am reminded about how lucky and grateful I am. Every time I hear mom talking on the phone about your story, at the end she always says, "Now he has been in remission for five years." Without you, I can't even imagine how life would be. Your drive and hunger to get your body healthy and out of that hospital bed has shown me how strong you really are, mentally, physically and emotionally. Your kindness and the amount of help and support you provide to people has inspired me to the maximum level. The things you have taught me in life about how to admit when I am wrong and how to treat other people (especially my mom when my phone was taken away) has helped me through school, hockey, friends, family, and everything that I have in my life. As I said, I couldn't even imagine a life without you. You are the main supporter of this family, and I am blessed to have you here today.

Today, I still do wonder though, what did kick cancer out of your body. Isagenix? Naaaaa. Medicine? Probably not. Laughing at Impractical Jokers? YA BABY!!!!

I love you tati boy,
Nick

Dear Dad,

When I was age six, I remember when you were diagnosed with cancer. At that time, I had no clue what that was but I knew I wouldn't be able to see you every day. After one month of not seeing you, I got in the car and drove to NYC to visit you in the hospital. The minute I saw you, I burst into tears because I couldn't believe what happened. You had lost your hair, you looked very weak and you couldn't play with me anymore.

After days and weeks of you still going back and forth to the hospital, I only thought one thing, "Am I going to lose my best friend?" As time went by, I got to visit you more. The minute Aunt Missy gave you her stem cells, I knew everything was going to be okay.

After eighteen months, I was so happy that you were finally okay after all. And there I was holding your hand when we left the hospital. I finally knew my best friend was back and better than ever. I am so grateful for everyone and everything that helped you get through all of that. Dad, I am so proud of you and I love you.

Love, Sarah

INTRODUCTION

Anyone with cancer remembers exactly how the "news" was delivered to them. For Marc, it was August 2, 2011: "Sir, I'm sorry to say that there is cancer in your body. I'm not sure what kind it is or how severe it is yet, but we are sure that there is cancer in you." It would ultimately be stage 4 Hodgkin's lymphoma. For Lisa, it was May 20, 2013: "I'm sorry, my dear, I don't have good news for you." That news would be a rare form of breast cancer, late-stage invasive lobular carcinoma. How did they break the news to you?

Unfortunately, we are not handed an instruction manual when we are handed the heart-shattering news. But our wish for you is that you use this book as the instruction manual to take back your life, your health, and your relationships and to live life with a deeper purpose and passion than you ever thought possible.

While none of us wanted to hear those words, the path we were to endure was clear. Fight cancer with all the determination, strength and faith we could muster up. Surround ourselves with people who could love and support us. Seek out the best medical treatment we could find. And throughout the journey try to keep a positive outlook. If that seems like a list of impossibility don't worry, *you're not alone.*

If you are currently going through treatment, we understand that it feels like a full-time job. If you have finished treatment, and all of a sudden you have a lot of time on your hands, we hear you. We felt the same way!

The people in your life care, love and support you, but they don't really understand what you are going through. And that's okay, *you're not alone.*

This book is designed for anyone who is going or has gone through a cancer battle and wants to harness the power of the cancer journey as a force for positive change. In each chapter, we share our unique transformation before, during and after cancer in seven core areas: body, mind, relationship, career, finance, spirituality and contribution.

You'll find important tools you can use to manage the confusion and anxiety. You may access your exclusive SBC Toolbox of bonus material at www.shinebeyondcancer.com/toolbox. Our hope is that you'll achieve clarity, strength, and purpose. No matter where you are on this quest through cancer, we will quarterback you through all aspects of your life so that you too live a vibrant, abundant life.

We have written this book from our hearts and our experiences in a way that is vulnerable and transparent. It might not always look pretty because it wasn't.

Cancer is a profound journey! We have said many times, we would never wish this disease on anyone, but we are grateful to have had the experience.

We would like to congratulate you on choosing this book. And now…it's time to shine…Shine Beyond Cancer!

Keep Shining,
Lisa and Marc

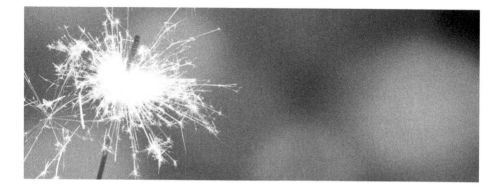

BODY

Natural forces within us are the true
healers of disease.

– Hippocrates, Father of Western Medicine

MARC'S BODY JOURNEY

MY BEGINNING

Who doesn't have body issues? Even without cancer, you may have wished your body was a different size or shape. But with cancer, maybe like me, you found your body was changing in ways you never anticipated. This is a behind the scenes look at how cancer took my body through the wringer. Hopefully, it will give you the realization that on the other side of cancer, your body is miraculously resilient.

I was a big boy: athletic, strong and competitive. Throughout high school, I was always active, and amongst my friends, I was considered to be the best athlete. Despite that, I still remember the feeling of embarrassment going school-clothes shopping with my mom and having to look for clothes in the husky department. These experiences created a lens that affected how I viewed myself physically in the future.

As an adult working in a stressful career, I knew I had to have the energy to show up every day and run my business. I wasn't strict with my nutrition, but I would try to avoid junk food as much as possible. I've never been a smoker and to this day I still can't stand the smell of cigarettes.

While I was a recreational drug user at the University of Albany, as were most of my peers, it never became a habit. During the 80s, a time when cocaine was rampant, I partook on the rare occasion but never as much as other coworkers. We would occasionally go out for drinks after work, but alcohol has never been a problem either. Overall, I listened to my body, enjoyed myself but never abused substances that could harm my body. The majority of the time I was making healthy lifestyle choices.

I tried my best to keep myself healthy all while maintaining a high-energy and fast-paced job as a broker on the floor of the New York Stock Exchange. I would never have predicted the twists and turns my body was going to take in the very near future.

MY FIRST HEALTH SCARE

It was August 1, 2006, and while there will be five more years before I hear the word "cancer" in conjunction with my body, at this time in my life I was under a mountain of stress from work. Up until then, I had an extremely successful business. I was making more money than I knew what to do with. I never dreamed of having the kind of life where I could live like a rockstar. Being a street kid from Brooklyn, this was a dream come true!

But change is inevitable. When computerization took over the New York Stock Exchange, my business seemingly dropped overnight. With eight employees, payroll taxes and a mountain of other business expenses, I was heading into what would prove to be a near deadly change in my body.

The large drop in income, an increase in business expenses and having to support a lifestyle that was unsustainable resulted in a stress-related heart attack.

I was on a fast pitch softball team with my uncle Steve, cousin Scott and one of my best friends, Dave Fox, in New Jersey, and it was one evening when disaster would strike. It was a hot and humid stretch in late July, and a few days prior to this game I wasn't feeling right. I was sweating profusely when I was outside, with little relief when I was in the air conditioning. I shrugged it off as weather-related discomfort until the Tuesday night when I was heading out to Jersey to play a game like I did every week. I could hardly keep up the walk with my friend to the PATH train, and I even asked to sit out an inning to stretch my chest, which I thought was pulled from a bad swing.

Feeling better, I hopped back in and finished out the game. Danielle, my wife, was there to drive me back to the city and had to stop three times on the NJ Turnpike so I could get out and stretch to relieve my chest pain. Fortunately, when we arrived home she insisted that I go to the hospital, much to my chagrin. I was only forty-three and I was healthy; what could possibly be wrong with me? The last thing on my mind was a heart attack, but I finally conceded and got in my friend Steve's car to head down to Beekman Hospital.

I walked into the hospital pretty calmly and started answering questions from the gentleman at the front desk. As we were speaking I saw that he was getting more and more concerned. He took me into a room and then administered an EKG. The next thing I knew, I was surrounded by eight doctors, multiple interns, and all the accompanying staff. I was watching them hook me up to machines and put all kinds of things into my body. Little did I know they were quietly talking amongst themselves about what steps to take to save my life. In minutes, I was loaded into an ambulance and transported from Beekman Hospital to New York-Presbyterian.

The team at New York-Presbyterian decided to put in stents. They recommended that we do the first one as soon as possible and the second one two weeks later. They knew my body would not handle having both stents put in at the same time.

Looking back on this time period now, it seems surreal. It's hard to believe it was just another experience in my life and not the wake-up call that it probably should have been for me. I was grateful to be on the mend physically and to be able to participate fully in the lives of my five children, whom I love very much.

Life went back to business as usual. I ate well and remained active for the most part, but not as diligently as I could have. I shifted gears and began working at my uncle and cousin's company in New York City, which was a nice change and a lot less pressure, but the problem was they partied like rockstars every night of the week.

As a father with two young children at the time, I would only agree to go out with them about once a week. I would choose a night where my family didn't really have anything going on and go party with them. I knew deep down though that I was abusing my body, and I couldn't afford another health crisis.

There were times when I was out late in Manhattan. I remember arriving home at 3:30 a.m. and then having to get up and go to work. I was still putting my body under more stress than was necessary, and I knew I wasn't making enough money at this job to feel secure. While I watched others grab fast food on the go, if possible I'd opt for a salad because I knew I could easily put on weight if I wasn't careful.

While I continued my routine over the next few years, the next health crisis appeared in January of 2011. Walking down a snowy concrete stairway headed to the gym, I slipped and fell down, landing on my iliac bone in my lower back. After collecting my suit, my duffle bag, my spilled coffee cup, and my pride, I headed to the shower to compose myself, lick my wounds and head to work. Never one to make a big deal of injuries, I walked it off during the day and laughed it off with my friends. But for the next six months, everyone noticed that my health took a turn for the worse.

THE DREADED CANCER DIAGNOSIS

After the fall, doctors diagnosed me with Epstein-Barr mononucleosis. I was told there was no protocol except patience. I lived with night sweats, weight loss and fatigue for the next several months. It got so bad that Danielle and I had to change our bed every morning because the sheets were just drenched. My once healthy skin lost its color and appeared an ashy gray. I was down roughly thirty-five pounds at this point and felt worse than ever. What happened to my once-strong and energetic body? I waited for the symptoms to subside, but it wasn't getting any better.

It was at this point when we all became afraid. Danielle was begging me to get a second opinion. My mother and mother-in-law were pestering

Danielle. And when you have three women telling you to do something, you eventually cave.

Not knowing what was wrong with me was the worst part. It couldn't be Epstein-Barr mono. I knew it had to be something else. We went back for another opinion and to be honest, when I finally got the diagnosis of stage 4 Hodgkin's lymphoma in August, eight months after the initial misdiagnosis, I felt relieved. Having a diagnosis meant that we finally had something we could effectively treat.

I'll never forget when the doctors and I sat down and they laid out the plan of action: twelve rounds of aggressive chemotherapy. For the next twenty-four weeks, I would undergo one week of chemo and then have one week off to recuperate. I had no idea what this would do to my body, but I was pretty sure it wasn't going to be pleasant.

At my weigh-in before my third round of chemo, the scale read 162 lbs. At more than thirty pounds down, I had lost twenty percent of my body weight and was way below my healthy set point. I looked in the mirror at my sunken cheekbones and my bony frame, and I couldn't imagine this downward spiral continuing much longer.

Emotionally I was a wreck. I had absolutely no energy to do things that once made me happy. I was taking three- or four-hour naps every day. I felt like the walking dead. I was at my lowest low. How could I endure losing my children? What about Danielle? I couldn't bear the thought of leaving her. The darkness surrounded me and all hope was seemingly lost. But often, the darkness is greatest before the dawn.

A TIME FOR CHANGE WAS UPON ME

During chemotherapy, I was attempting to eat anything and everything Danielle prepared for me. From shots of wheatgrass to organic peanut butter to spoonfuls of coconut oil, I was focused on using the right food to help my body heal. We attempted to get nutritional advice from the staff at the hospital but all they offered was a visit with the hospital nutritionist. We were told to follow the old, outdated, antiquated American food pyramid that no one follows anymore. Danielle and I blew off that advice and knew it was our job to figure the nutritional part out on our own. I was eating a lot of food with dense calories, but nothing was sticking on my body. We were trying our best but our best wasn't enough. Finally, in a moment of desperation, Danielle called our friend Lisa DeMayo, crying and wondering what else we could do.

> **Focusing on happiness changed things for my body, and for my mind.**

Lisa had just discovered an organic, high protein nutrition company and thought it might work for us. We were willing to do anything, so we said YES and had a box full of food shipped to us immediately. I started the high-protein diet right away and within days my energy was on the upswing. I felt a peace come over me, and my body started to regain weight. I noticed my muscle mass returning. In the following few weeks, I was able to start coaching my son's basketball team again and I no longer needed hours a day to nap. Was this part of the answer? I sure hoped so!

While it might sound crazy, I did lots of laughing, smiling and watching funny TV shows, like "The Impractical Jokers," to will myself to get better. Laughing changed the endorphins in my brain and promoted healing. It relieved my stress to create an environment that was conducive to recovery. Focusing on happiness changed things for my body, and for my mind.

Starting the fourth round of chemo, I was feeling entirely better. I was putting weight back on and through the twelfth round, my energy was continuing to get better and the doctors were impressed with my progress.

Towards the end of chemo, I had a PET scan. I was hopeful that the cancer was gone and I would be given a clean bill of health. After all, statistics show that eighty percent of people with my type of cancer recover fully. Unfortunately, that was not the case for me. With the disappointing results, unbeknownst to me, the oncology team had already planned to do a stem cell transplant. So, for the next three weeks I was told to take an experimental chemotherapy pill and when that finished they took another PET scan. That scan brought more awful news.

My cancer was worse than it was when I was diagnosed. I felt discouraged but I had confidence that the doctors would find the right solution. They cut the pill off immediately and ordered a third IV type of chemo. After that, I was scheduled to have a stem cell transplant. Having endured so much already, I was sure I could handle this too, but much to my dismay, it was the toughest round yet.

I was hospital-ridden for five straight days of a continuous IV drip. I was away from my kids, away from my wife and having to live with all the protocols of a hospital. From the bed automatically moving every twenty minutes, to the nursing staff checking my vitals every few hours, to declining the horrible hospital food and trying to sleep only to be awakened by the next doctor or janitor, it was a living nightmare. Although I was never really nauseous, I was drained...and bald. Luckily, after it was over I was sent home to recover for five days. This same cycle repeated six times, so the next two months would be my worst to date. Would this be the solution? I prayed it would be.

My prayers were answered. Chemo round three basically worked, except for one spot. My iliac bone. The spot where I had landed on that fateful day almost two years ago, was still causing lingering problems. My team of doctors told me that they were unable to do the stem cell transplant until they got rid of that spot. Their plan for me was to undergo twenty-one rounds of radiation therapy. For me, this involved staying away from my family even more. The treatments were located one hundred miles from home, and it wasn't practical to go back and forth every day. Fortunately, a childhood friend, David Rosen let me crash at his apartment multiple times every week, and during breaks, I'd drive the two hours home only to return twenty-four hours later.

Thankfully, the radiation treatment knocked out the cancer in my iliac bone, and in November of 2012 I received stem cells from my sister, Melissa, and underwent the procedure. The five-hour drip was easy, but the five days of poisonous chemo before that was the worst part. The oncologists had to completely kill my immune system in order to rebuild it again.

Was this the light at the end of the tunnel? Would I soon be cancer-free?

I continued to do everything I could to make myself smile and be happy. I would go for short walks outside just to get fresh air and take in the smells of New Jersey in November and December.

Between the laughter, the nutrition plan, the chemo, the radiation therapy, and the stem cell transplant, miracles started happening in my body and eventually knocked out the cancer.

FINALLY, CANCER-FREE

I am grateful to say that I am six years cancer-free. I am back to my ideal body weight and have the energy to run my own online business and parent two teenagers and three adult daughters who reside in Arizona. It's been such a joy to watch Samantha, DJ and Brittany launch thriving careers, and I even had the privilege of walking my oldest, Samantha, down the aisle last year. There wasn't a dry eye in the venue. Including mine.

To this day, I still follow the same nutrition program and have incorporated some of their athletic and performance products into my workout routine. It's been seven years, and I firmly believe that it changed the trajectory of my recovery at a time when things weren't looking so good.

I exercise five days a week and continue to stay active. I play softball, walk the beach with my wife, go to Power Plate at Lisa Dimond's wellness studio and have enjoyed CrossFit, yoga and boxing. I'm grateful to have relocated to Naples, Florida, which has been voted to be the healthiest and happiest city in the country. This move was one of the best things we did as a family. There are lots of options here for me to try new things and continue to stay active and healthy.

MY INSIGHT AND ENCOURAGEMENT

Whether you are going through treatments or you're cancer-free, I want to offer a suggestion: experiment on your own body when it comes to nutrition and fitness. There is something that is going to work perfectly for you. Remember, the things that worked for me may not work for you, but if you want more details on the specifics of what I did, I am happy to help you. Feel free to reach out to me on our Shine Beyond Cancer Facebook page.

You have nothing to lose when you try new things. If what you are doing today is not working, find something else. It's not going to work tomorrow or the next day if it's not working already.

Your mind and your body are connected, even more than you

> **Experiment on your own body when it comes to nutrition and fitness. There is something that is going to work perfectly for you.**

think; and monitoring your thoughts is crucial. We'll talk about that in the Mindset section of the book. So go out there on a personal scavenger hunt and find the things that will work for you to sustain you during your cancer treatments and repair your body. I believe you can be cancer-free and even improve your body beyond where it was when you received your diagnosis. Let cancer be your gift to change your body. It has been mine.

LISA'S BODY JOURNEY

BEFORE CANCER

Before hearing the terrifying news that I had cancer in May of 2013, I was in the best shape of my life. At 128 pounds, I felt great about my rock-solid body and was feeling healthy and strong. I had been introduced to Power Plate, whole-body vibration training, by a dear friend of mine in 2009. When I started personal training sessions soon thereafter, I became thoroughly addicted. My thirty-minute workouts worked for me, and I felt at the top of my game. The health benefits are pretty awesome too! In addition to the natural neuromuscular response and thirty to forty involuntary muscle contractions per second, Power Plate stimulates the lymphatic system, reduces cortisol (a stress hormone) levels and increases circulation.

It was in July of 2012 that I realized I really wanted to be a part of this world. I made it my goal to open my own Power Plate studio to bring awareness of what it can do for people. So I got all the certifications I needed for Power Plate, including my personal training certification from the National Academy of Sports Medicine. I was so excited about this new venture and opened the doors to my own personal training business in February 2013. My future was looking bright, but there was something in my body that wasn't quite right.

DISCOVERY

In December 2012, I noticed a hard spot on my left breast. It wasn't actually a round lump and it didn't feel like a pea. I mentioned it to a friend who was a nurse. She took a look and thought it could be a calcium deposit or my implant could be encapsulated.

At the time, I was busy helping a woman who I considered to be my surrogate mother. I made a mental note to have the hardness in my left breast checked out by the plastic surgeon who had put in my implants eight years earlier. Fate intervened and the woman I was assisting got very sick. She was diagnosed with non-Hodgkin's lymphoma. We spent eleven days in the hospital and set up hospice, so she'd be more comfortable at home. She passed away six days later on Christmas Eve. Those seventeen days were some of the most difficult, emotional days I've ever experienced. I had lost yet another person so dear to my heart. Over the next week, I barely left my house because I was so devastated and grieving deeply.

On January 1, 2013, I woke up early, felt grateful for a new year and declared to myself it was going to be my best year ever. Having just witnessed a vibrant woman pass away in seventeen days, I was reminded that life is short. 2013 was going to be the year where I finally did what I wanted to do: get my personal training certification and open a studio. Between grieving and meeting the world with a new attitude, I forgot about the hardness in my breast.

By March 2013, I was on my way. I had a clear vision and was excited about life. In two months, I went from 0 to twenty-three clients. I loved helping people achieve their goals. In March 2013, I celebrated my forty-eighth birthday by going hang gliding. In the same month, I made an appointment with my plastic surgeon to have my implants checked and get a mammogram. The next available appointment was May 8.

THE ROLLER COASTER RIDE BEGINS

On May 8, 2013, in the late afternoon, I eagerly went to my doctor appointment. The doctor and I sat in his office and talked. I explained the hardness that I felt and where it was. He agreed that it sounded like an encapsulated implant. When he examined me and felt the hardness, he looked me in the eye and said, "That is not your implant." He turned to the nurse and said, "Order a mammogram and ultrasound. STAT!" I thought to myself, *STAT? Isn't that what doctors say when someone is dying?*

We all know that waiting to do a medical test can take days and even weeks. Not so when the doctor orders a test STAT. My doctor appointment was three p.m. on a Wednesday. My mammogram and ultrasound were scheduled at 8:20 the next morning.

Buckle up…it's going to be a bumpy ride.

Why is it always 32° F in medical offices and testing facilities? I learned on day one to dress warm and take a sweater. I checked in, filled out the stack of forms that unbeknownst to me was going to become a routine drill many times over, and waited. Waiting is the worst part, especially for those who are patience-challenged. I heard my name called, "Lisa Dimond!"

I was taken to a tiny cubicle, nicely appointed to make it feel homey, handed a gown and asked to strip waist up. And then more waiting. Finally, I was directed to take my mammogram. This machine was obviously designed by a man.

Part one was over. Back to the cubicle, I went to wait for the ultrasound tech. Thirty-five minutes passed. Off to the ultrasound room. "Wow," the technician said. *This cannot be good*, I thought.

"Is everything okay?" I asked.

"This is really big," she replied, and she was not talking about my breast.

Part two was over. I dressed and waited for the radiologist to read the results. The room was dark and I was scared to death.

The results finally came in. I followed the tech down the very sterile hallway to what looked like a high-tech computer lab. The only lights were from computer screens displaying black, white and gray images of what I assumed were my breasts. I don't even remember what the radiologist looked like, but he said to me that nothing was detected on the mammogram. *Ahhh, home free!!! NOT!*

After a long pause, he explained to me that a very large mass showed up on the ultrasound. "I cannot rule out cancer." He continued to talk and point at the images, but I didn't hear a word he said. He handed me a yellow piece of paper, still talking to me, but I still couldn't hear him at all. He had me at "I cannot rule out cancer." There was an awkward pause, and I realized at that point that I was supposed to leave but I couldn't move. Why didn't he have me sit down in a chair? I felt like I was going to throw up. "Do you have any questions?" he asked.

My mind was reeling. The only thing I could come up with was, "What am I supposed to do now?"

He pointed to the bottom of the yellow sheet and said, "You need to contact a breast surgeon."

I absently said, "Thank you." I do not remember leaving that building, getting in my car or driving home.

After I arrived home, I sent a text to a very dear friend of mine who is a radiation oncologist in Ft. Myers. "Can you recommend a breast surgeon?"

Ten seconds later, my phone rang. It was him. "Why?" he asked. I told him what I knew. He gave me the number of a friend of ours in Naples, also a radiation oncologist. Before I even had a chance to dial the number, the Naples doctor called me. He gave me the name and number of a breast surgeon; I called and made an appointment. The first available appointment was in ten days. Ten days? Do I even have ten days to wait?

I quickly realized that it pays to have a friend who is an oncologist. From that point forward, he took over making appointments and getting results

"STAT." It was a Thursday. My breast surgeon appointment got bumped up to the following Monday, May 13, 2013. My biopsy was scheduled for Thursday, May 16. The results were in on May 20, 2013.

"I'm sorry, my dear. I don't have good news." When the doctor entered the room, those were his first words to me. I asked him to double-check that he was in the right room. There had been another woman in the waiting room with me earlier. Maybe, I was hoping, he had her chart instead of mine. He did actually check. He was in the correct room. I know I was there in that room for at least another thirty minutes, though I do not remember another word he said.

The next thing I remember was sitting in my car in the parking lot. I was angry and yelling at the top of my lungs, "Are you fucking kidding me? Why?" over and over again. And then I thought, how am I going to tell the few friends who knew that I was at that appointment? And then I cried…how was I going to tell my two beautiful daughters, ages fifteen and eighteen at the time? My heart was broken.

Once you know you have cancer, a series of tests and doctor appointments ensue. MRI, PET scan, blood tests. And then…just when you get your head wrapped around it…there is more.

I began taking a friend with me to my appointments with a pen and notebook. The ultrasound showed a mass measuring 4.2 cm. OK. The MRI showed 5.4 cm. It had grown in just a few weeks. The PET scan, which lights up cancer cells like a Christmas tree, was done from my neck to my pelvis to determine if it had spread from my left breast to any other part of my body. Again, the waiting for results was the worst. GOOD NEWS! It was contained in the left breast.

At this point, only a handful of close friends knew. I made a decision to hold off telling my daughters until I knew exactly what I was dealing with and what the treatment plan was going to be. I did not want them to suffer through the roller coaster ride of testing and waiting. My fear was like a weight that I lugged around with me.

THE TREATMENT PLAN

"My Team" now consisted of a breast surgeon, radiation oncologist (my friend) and a medical oncologist. The plan was surgery and chemotherapy. Radiation was a possibility. Anyone who knows me will tell you that I am a control freak. This stage was when I started to take control of my own healing from all aspects: mind, body, and soul. This was the day I became a research fanatic. I began to research natural, holistic and complementary alternatives.

Healing became my full-time job! As I began my own regimen of diet, supplements, meditation, oxygen therapy and exercise, the doctors put their own regimen in place. I wasn't so sure about theirs and decided to seek a second opinion from another breast surgeon. Guided by my strength, courage and intuition, I went with the second opinion. Finally, I had all three doctors on the same page with the following plan:

1. Bilateral double mastectomy with lymph node dissection

2. Aggressive chemotherapy

3. Radiation, if necessary

THE MOST DIFFICULT DAY

As difficult as some days were during that year, there is one single day that will forever stand out: the day I told my daughters. I didn't really prepare for that moment. The words came from my heart and I knew if they saw my strength, courage, and grace they would find it for themselves as well. They sat in adirondack chairs on the lanai, and I sat on the floor between them. I took their hands and said, "There is no easy way to say what I am about to say, so I am just going to say it. I have been diagnosed with breast cancer." Tears began to stream down their beautiful faces. My heart was breaking. "But we are going to get through this with strength, courage, and grace. We are going to have good days and bad, but I'm pretty sure mostly good. And when we feel like crying, we are going to cry. And when it is all over, there won't be anything the three of us can't handle!"

And then the battery of questions came (they are my girls after all), the most important and most difficult from my fifteen-year-old, Olivia. "Are you going to die?"

My response was immediate and firm. "No! Not from this!" I replied. And it was at that moment that I knew I wasn't!

The night before my surgery, I took my girls out to dinner and watched the sunset at La Playa, which is my favorite spot on the beach. I didn't want to leave the beach that night. I knew once I left that spot that I was on a path that was littered with uncertainty. But I knew I wasn't going to give up. They were the inspiration for the hard-fought battle.

TREATMENT

In June of 2013, prior to my scheduled breast surgery, I consulted with a plastic surgeon. Based on the imaging results, the breast surgeon gave me the options of lumpectomy, single mastectomy or double mastectomy. Based on my consultation with the plastic surgeon, I chose double mastectomy because he explained that it is nearly impossible to reconstruct just one breast and have it match the existing breast.

On June 21, 2013, one month after the diagnosis and battery of tests, I had my surgery. With my daughters and one of my best friends, Louise, by my side, I arrived at the hospital in the early morning. I was most definitely filled with anxiety but my spirits were high. The surgeon entered the pre-op room and explained once again the procedure. They will biopsy a lymph node during surgery. She explained that I would have at least two drains when I woke up. If there was a third drain, the lymph node will be positive and they will have removed my lymph nodes on the left side. Sure enough, there were three drains! Are you kidding me? I was devastated. I cried, I sobbed and for the first time during this process, I just broke down.

My surgery was on a Friday. I went home Saturday morning. I never took another pain pill after leaving the hospital that day, and I was more determined than ever that this was not going to control my life. Saturday afternoon was my first visit from the home health care nurse to change the bandages on my chest. She asked if I wanted to see my chest. I wasn't ready. Saturday evening, I went with friends for a sunset boat ride and had a cookout at my home to celebrate getting through surgery. Sunday, after going to the movies with my daughters, I went home to meet my home health care nurse again. She asked me again if I wanted to see my changes. I still wasn't ready. I trained all of my scheduled clients on Monday. I never missed a day of training my clients during my entire treatment.

For the five days following surgery, the home health care nurse came to change the bandages and she always asked if I wanted to see it. I always said, "No, thanks." However, on the last day she came, I knew I would have to learn to change the bandages myself. That meant I had to look at my chest and do it myself.

No longer could I close my eyes and ignore the drastic changes as if the whole thing hadn't happened. I looked in the mirror and told myself, *it is what it is.* When I saw the changes from the surgery, surprisingly I didn't feel like it was gross or horrible. I breathed a sigh of relief and accepted that it was simply a change.

SURGERY FOLLOW-UP

During my appointment following my surgery, I learned that the tumor on the left was nine centimeters and the cancer had spread to the right breast. The tumor on the right was one centimeter. The surgeons removed all but a few lymph nodes on the left. The majority of the lymph nodes tested positive. Yes, this was aggressive. In just one month, it had doubled and spread. Chemo would now be more aggressive and radiation was a must. I was told that I would also need a hysterectomy after treatment. *WHAT?* I was at stage 3B, which is one step from stage 4.

The next day, I got a call from the radiation oncologist informing me that I'd been scheduled for an MRI of the brain. *WHAT?* He explained to me that the type of cancer I had commonly spreads to the brain. It had to be checked out. I thought breast cancer was breast cancer. I discovered that I also had invasive lobular carcinoma.

My research showed that this type of breast cancer is 1) rare (occurs in only ten percent of all breast cancer cases) and 2) aggressive. This was the first time I researched survival rates. I never felt that I was going to die from this, but I needed to know what I was up against. The survival rate for my stage is thirty-six percent. Once again, I wrapped my head around it and said to myself, OK, game on!

I went to my brain MRI appointment alone. I made a deal with God that day in the waiting room. *Dear God, if there is some chance you can spare me from brain cancer, I will fight my ass off to beat the breast cancer and I will do good things to help others going through this!!! Please!!!* I knew I was strong but wasn't sure I was brain cancer strong.

My doctor assured me I would have the results the same day. After the MRI, friends gathered at my house to be with me when the news came. We waited an awkward two hours and it felt like an eternity. The phone finally rang, but I was afraid to answer it. When I did, my doctor had great news: my brain was all clear. *Thank you, God!*

From that point forward, I knew I was not going to die. I had a fight ahead of me but I was ready. I was strong, healthy and positive. I was going to do this with strength, courage, and grace.

I healed beautifully from the surgery.

CHEMOTHERAPY

Step 1) Another surgery. I was told I had to have a mediport placed in my chest. A mediport is a catheter that connects the port to a vein. Under the skin, the port has a septum through which drugs can be injected and blood samples can be drawn many times. This required outpatient surgery. There are two risks; a one in a hundred chance that the doctors could puncture the lung during surgery and the risk of infection. Of course, I researched this and discovered that people have died from an infection with a mediport. Note to self, this was not going to happen to me. Punctured lung? Yep, this did happen to me but I recovered quickly and was able to leave the hospital fourteen hours later even though they admitted me to an overnight stay.

Step 2) Chemo treatments. I was told the doctors were pulling out the "big guns" for my chemo regimen. I received the three most aggressive, toxic drugs on the market. My first treatment was on July 17, 2013.

I educated myself on chemotherapy and informed family, friends and doctors that I would not be one of the statistics. I was doing this my way.

I received treatments every other Wednesday for three to five hours. My daughters and friends took turns sitting with me during that time. There were moments when I longed for my normal, healthy, carefree life, but I mostly meditated and listened to positive affirmations to stay in the moment and focused on the fight.

I was successful getting through chemo with no real side effects other than losing my hair. Family, friends, doctors, and nurses were amazed at my healthy blood readings and my energy. I was able to maintain both my white and red blood cell counts, which I managed through eating an alkaline diet. Chemotherapy often causes one to lose the sense of taste, and with that, many people also lose their appetite, which causes weight loss. I, on the other hand, did not lose or gain an ounce and worked very hard at that. I was 128 pounds at the start and I was 128 pounds at the end. The doctors couldn't believe it. They told me to keep doing whatever it was I was doing.

I researched my own nutrition and supplements, and I knew what I needed to keep my immune system boosting higher. I think that helped me with the side effects of chemo. Also, I was on vibration and stimulated my lymphatic system every day. I moved my body, which helped immensely. When most people get their diagnosis and hear the side effects, they choose to go home and sit on the couch to manifest the side effects. Those side effects are real, but I firmly believe that moving my body every day, whether I wanted to or not, was critical to staying healthy through the treatments.

I was working, I was on a nutritional plan that was keeping my counts up and I also did acupuncture once a week. This was going on along with an aggressive chemo plan. Most people get chemo and then get two weeks off to recover. They call these recovery weeks. There were no recovery weeks for me. I always turned to acupuncture the day after chemo, which helped to boost my immune system. I didn't believe I was a victim to cancer. I focused on the future and what I had to do to make it happen the way I wanted. I learned to celebrate the victories no matter how big or small.

I remained on my positive path and received my final chemo treatment on October 31, 2013. I had learned that the staff and nurses were dressing up that day in superhero costumes. Very appropriate! They are superheros, and I am still grateful for their care and compassion. I dressed up that day as well…full blown Catwoman!

A DAY OF UNCONDITIONAL LOVE AND SUPPORT

I started to lose my long, beautiful, blonde hair right after my second treatment, July 31, 2013. I didn't tell anyone and gave myself a couple of days to "wrap my head around it." Anyone who knows me knows I will look for any excuse to throw a party. As a matter of fact, I regularly threw a Sunday Funday cookout at my house. On any given Sunday, there could be fifteen to thirty people at my house.

On Friday, August 2, 2013, I announced to my daughters and friends that on Sunday, August 4, I was throwing a "No Hair Affair" and would be shaving my head poolside. I asked friends to bring hats and scarves that I could wear until I got through this. The party started as usual. When

I announced it was time to shave my head, one of my friends stepped up and said, "I'm going first!" *WHAT???* I was blown away. Seven of my friends shaved their heads that day. I felt so much love and support! My anxiety faded. My daughters and I knew we weren't alone. My friends gave me the gift of strength, courage, and grace to keep going that day.

When the evening was over, the girls and I cleaned up a little bit and it was finally time to see myself. I walked into the bathroom and lifted my eyes to the mirror and started sobbing. Some of the tears were for vanity, some just sadness but being bald made me feel stronger. It became part of the fighting armor that would get me through this fight. A lot of the time, I didn't even wear a hat or bandana; I just rocked bald.

NEXT STOP—RADIATION

I had a two-week vacation from treatment. I began radiation on November 15, 2013, every day, Monday through Friday, for thirty-three treatments. During my two week break, I researched radiation, the effects and ways to prevent them from happening to me. Skin toxicity! No, this was not going to happen to me.

Although my treatments only took ten minutes, my own natural preventative treatments would take forty to sixty minutes each day after the treatment. I never did experience skin toxicity. However, with only a couple of weeks to go, the fight began to take its toll. I was having a difficult time sleeping and became exhausted. That was when I dug a little deeper and kept going.

My final treatment was January 14, 2014. My journal entry that day reads, "Today is the day!!! The end of a very profound and successful fight. Way to go, girl!!!"

I brought in cupcakes and balloons on my last treatment day. The radiation techs and staff went outside with me and we each released a balloon—a symbol for me that I was releasing the past and very much looking forward to the future. A CT scan had confirmed I was cancer free!

CANCER FREE BUT NOT HOME FREE

In July 2014, I went to my OB-GYN for my annual exam. Two days later, I got a phone call: "You have an abnormal pap result." *WHAT?* I had a biopsy the next week and sure enough, precancerous.

At that point, I was given two options: keep an eye on it or hysterectomy. "I'll take the hysterectomy, please." So here we were again, another surgery. Of course, there were risks but the procedure was fairly simple. I woke up from surgery and was told that my bladder was punctured during the procedure. Turns out it wasn't as simple as the doctor had thought. They had to place a catheter as well because of the punctured bladder. I was told, it could take two to four weeks before the bladder healed, and six to eight weeks of recovery for the hysterectomy. My surgery was on a Friday. I went home on Saturday morning. I went to my studio (catheter and all) on Monday and continued to train my clients through the entire recovery process.

Almost a year after my last radiation treatment, January 1, 2015, I developed a cellulitis infection in the radiation site of my chest on the left side. The doctor put me on antibiotics. When I came off the antibiotics, I got shingles on the left side of my face. While I was still on medication for the shingles, I spiked a fever of 104° F. On February 1, 2015, I went to the emergency room. Because I was a cancer patient, they ran every test possible. Even with all the scans and blood they took, they couldn't find anything so they prescribed a general antibiotic and sent me home.

Three days later, my fever spiked again but this time it was 105° F. I went to my primary care doctor, and she pulled my file and hospital records. It turned out I had *E. coli* in my bloodstream, and it had gone to the lining of my heart. It was terrifying! I could barely breathe, and there was massive pain on the left side of my chest.

My primary doctor sent me straight to the hospital. I ended up staying in the hospital for almost a month. I became septic and I almost died. In the hospital, I was on massive doses of several different antibiotics. When they did release me, I left with a PICC (peripherally inserted central catheter) line in my arm and had to do daily infusions at the infectious disease doctor's office. I did that for four weeks and was on an oral antibiotic for four weeks after that.

After that experience, I felt like hell! I had chronic fatigue, the inside of my chest was inflamed and daily life became painful. Showering felt like having darts hitting my chest from the water. This went on for the next two years, and it was probably one of the worst points in my life.

My active, energetic, enthusiastic life came to a screeching halt throughout those two years. I would go to my studio and put all my energy into my clients, and when I left at the end of the day I went straight home and went to bed. Everything I ate went right through me because I had an overgrowth of bad bacteria, known as Candida, from all of the antibiotics. I suffered through chronic bloating and rashes all over my body.

I remember having to sleep in long sleeves because I would wake up in the middle of the night scratching myself to the point of bleeding. I couldn't find relief anywhere! I spent a lot of money looking for something, anything, that would make me feel good. My oncologist was trained to help treat cancer and really nothing else, so I felt like I was on my own to figure this out. I would go in to get checked out periodically because once you have had cancer you're never out of the woods. No matter how many times I asked, there was nothing they could do for me beyond making sure I didn't have cancer again.

2017 BRINGS RELIEF

Throughout 2015 and most of 2016, I struggled to find something to combat the stress that was coursing through my body: emotional stress from not feeling well, distress of being sick and having cancer, and toxic stress from chemo, radiation and antibiotics. I would learn that my liver was functioning at only thirty-five percent, and my body was shutting down organ by organ.

It was a crazy feeling because you don't truly appreciate your health until you don't have it anymore. It was May 2016 (three years post-diagnosis) that I met Marc and Danielle. Marc walked into my studio to try a different form of exercise (and I am so grateful for that day). He had heard about Power Plate at a Tony Robbins event. (Thank you, Tony Robbins.) We instantly had a connection—the connection that only fellow cancer survivors feel. He signed up to train at the studio and little did I know that our meeting would be the start of so much more.

Marc and Danielle were not just clients—we became friends, the kind of friends that feel like family. As Marc shared his cancer experience with me and his superfood nutrition plan that kept his body in optimal fight mode, I knew I needed to try it. In August 2016, I received my first box of supplements and I noticed that my energy was returning. I had less bloating and better mental clarity (super important for chemo brain). My body was starting to make a comeback, but I was still struggling with the liver issue and the daily discomfort I felt on the left side of my chest.

> For me, my breasts don't define who I am and neither does cancer. Cancer doesn't define my life. It gives me a better definition of my life.

Since radiation kills everything, I literally had no blood flow in my left chest wall. Because of this, I was not a candidate for reconstruction. There wasn't a plastic surgeon who would operate on me because they thought it either wouldn't take or I would get an infection due to the lack of blood flow.

I was considering hyperbaric chamber treatments, but it was time-consuming and very expensive. Toward the end of 2016, I was introduced, by a dear friend, to a medical device that stimulates the microcirculation system. Literally, within five days of using this device, I could tell good things were happening in my body. I purchased my own device in January 2017 and began incorporating it into my daily healing routine.

I'm happy to report that there is no longer inflammation in my chest and my energy levels have gone off the charts. My liver is functioning at one hundred percent. That device, coupled with Marc's superfood nutrition, changed my life. Things that used to take me a month to accomplish when I was sick, I now can get done in a day. It really has given me my life back, and I have been cleared for reconstruction! My kids have their mom back, my clients have their trainer back and everything about my life is better.

CLOSING THOUGHTS

At the writing of this book, I am five years post-diagnosis. I went through treatment and the aftermath of post-treatment complications that nearly ended my story. I am here and alive, and I have never felt better. My views on my body have certainly changed as well as my outlook.

So far, and even though I am a candidate now, I have opted against getting reconstruction. It's a personal choice, and it doesn't bother me not having breasts. It certainly hasn't stopped me from doing everything I want. I did, however, have a tough moment recently.

Before cancer, my breasts were great! I had a whole closet full of cute tops and clothes, which I can't wear now because I don't have breasts to fill them out properly. I was in Nordstrom searching for an outfit to wear to an upcoming event and I couldn't find anything that worked for me. Right across the aisle was the lingerie department. I knew that Nordstrom has a mastectomy department so I walked over and asked the salesperson if she could help me.

This process turned out to be extremely uncomfortable. Imagine a young woman, no more than twenty-two years old, seeing you naked with no breasts! And she even stayed in the dressing room with me while I figured out how everything worked.

I made a quick decision and bought the prosthesis and a bra, and my total was nearly $800! I never thought about buying boobs at Nordstrom, and I certainly didn't plan to do it that day, but as I walked out of the store with my new boobs in the bag, I began to cry.

By the time I reached my car, I was sobbing. I realized I had never really dealt with the loss of my breasts. I had great boobs and a pretty perfect body before, and now it's pretty imperfect. I am learning to be okay with that. I grieved for the things that had changed, and it felt good to cry and get it out. It felt like I was blessing myself and loving myself and accepting my new normal.

For me, my breasts don't define who I am and neither does cancer. Cancer doesn't define my life. It gives me a better definition of my life. My advice to you, no matter where you are in your cancer journey, is to allow yourself to grieve the changes, love yourself and embrace who you really are.

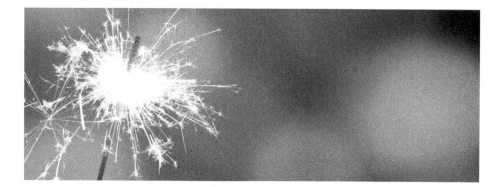

MINDSET

I am not what happened to me. I am
what I choose to become.

– *Carl Jung*

MARC'S MINDSET TRANSFORMATION

CHANGE

Buddha once said, "The secret of health for both mind and body is not to mourn for the past, or to worry about the future, but to live in the present moment wisely and earnestly," and I believe it's true. The mind is an amazing thing, and it will take you exactly where you don't want to be if you are not careful. It's normal to have times where you want to give up, to say "fuck it" or to ask, "why me?" How do I know? That was how I felt at times! We are human, and it's okay to have those thoughts once in a while. The trick is to recognize when your mind is heading down that road and correct course as soon as humanly possible.

Thank God that one year prior to my diagnosis, I was fortunate enough to begin to change the way I thought. Before that, I would have described myself as high-strung, anxious and hot-tempered. The fast pace and in-your-face lifestyle of New York City had rubbed off on me, and I became the stereotypical New Yorker. Along with that, I was a major worrier. My parents are champion worriers, and it has gotten much worse as they've gotten older. At times, it was totally overwhelming! All of my life, I grew up completely unaware of personal development, self-help and the power of positive thinking. You truly don't know what you don't know. It was by a stroke of luck that I was presented with an opportunity to change my outlook.

WHEN THINGS STARTED TO SHIFT

Looking back at the first half of 2010 I realize that's when I hit my mental rock bottom. It had been three and a half years since we closed our NYSE business and I still could not find a path to professional fulfillment. I started day trading, working on a desk as a sales trader and a research salesman.

I expected these positions to be an easy transition with my twenty-five years of knowledge in the financial industry. However, none of these experiences were financially fruitful or mentally stimulating. Add on top of that a two-hour commute each way which is enough in itself to drive someone crazy!

Cancer doesn't define you, cancer is just a part of your story. Guard your mind and make it work for you, not against you.

When we moved from NYC out to NJ, we moved into a gorgeous home on the water that we had built four and a half years earlier in partnership with my in-laws when times were good. We had somewhere to call home and my kids had the pleasure of living with their grandparents for the next six years. However, for me, I missed the hustle and bustle of living in Tribeca, and I resented the long commute every moment.

My mood had been declining for the last four years, and I was not in a good place at all. I couldn't see how down I truly was.

Fortunately, my ambitious wife, Danielle, was in a much better place. Because of her new career as a virtual franchise owner, she was exposed to a lot of personal growth experiences and events. She read and studied from the best in personal development, like Tony Robbins, Jim Rohn, Brian Tracy, and others. Danielle always encouraged me to join her, but I thought I knew better. I assumed I could get through all of this by myself, but I was wrong. I was sinking lower and lower into depression and then finally by the grace of God something happened.

The phone rang and it was Wendy, my first cousin, inviting me to attend a four-day transformational workshop. She raved about how amazing it was and how much she learned. She was completely sold on her new mindset and wanted to share it with me. I figured that if it was good enough for her, then it was good enough for me too and I would give it a try. I decided to take a chance, on me.

I hate to admit it, but my attitude going into the basic workshop was dismal. I remember asking myself, "What the hell am I thinking?" Fortunately, I wasn't the only one. Next to me was an open seat, and at two minutes to seven a girl came rushing in and sat down. She looked at me and said, "What the fuck are we doing here?!" Allison, a tough girl from Brooklyn, brought a smile to my face and together we laughed.

All I can say is that after the four days were over, I went and signed up for the advanced course right away. There were fifty-four people in this advanced workshop, and I had the opportunity to meet an amazing variety of people, from every walk of life. In this workshop, I met and befriended a woman who has become my personal confidant. She knows so much about me and has become one of my dearest friends in my life. Fran Peltz and I were meant to cross paths.

What I learned had changed my mindset, and I understood things about myself that I had never seen before. I saw that I was capable of so much more than I was doing and that the universe was an abundant place supporting me at every turn. After the five-day advanced course ended, I was all in!

I signed up for the three-month leadership program that provided accountability in six different areas. I learned to set and achieve goals through our weekly meetings and coaching calls, and at the end of the three months, I had a completely new outlook on how my life was going to take shape moving forward. I was hopeful again and regained the drive and determination that I had lost over the last few years.

Now, I wanted to pay it forward and agreed to volunteer coach the advanced course students. I saw them transform. The work really took people from living a routine, humdrum life to thriving again. They were setting goals and making plans to maximize their gifts and talents. All of these experiences put me in a completely different mindset, and thank God because I had no idea what was coming in the near future. These tools would be put to the test. The eight months I had invested in this program was invaluable. It was an amazing experience with phenomenal people who have remained my truest friends. The entire coaching program and the experiences I had while in the workshops completely turned me around. These programs made me realize that the universe has a plan.

THEN WHAT?

Adversity and disappointment had no place in my life anymore. God had a plan, and I was confident that I could handle anything that would come my way. Little did I know this new program was going to be tested! My fall and health decline would put my newly cultivated skills into action. Would they work, would they not work? Even though I was "all in" and had seen many transformations, including my own, my mind was still messing with me. I started to get sick shortly after all these courses completed, and I struggled to use these new tools to get through it. Many days were hard; I didn't know what was wrong with me and it was frustrating. I was exercising my new muscles of positivity and gratitude, and at times I was just plain exhausted.

DIAGNOSIS, FINALLY

When the doctors finally determined I had stage 4 Hodgkin's lymphoma, a wave of relief washed over me. Hearing the word cancer to most people is a death sentence, but as crazy as that sounds, to me it was a way to target my thoughts towards healing. It was going from unknown to known. Finally, with a diagnosis, a strategic plan to better health was on the horizon. And I had Danielle, who was and still is my number one supporter and cheerleader. She had also just completed the transformational program with me and was in a similar mindset. We had the knowledge and the tools we needed; now we just needed to follow the plan.

THE NEXT STEPS

After the initial diagnosis, we picked a doctor and hospital that fit our plan. The doctor we chose was highly recommended by three separate friends who did not know each other. It was like a piece of God's puzzle coming together.

Throughout treatment, there were times I felt defeated, especially during the first round of chemotherapy. Maybe you have felt that way too? Rest assured, it's normal to have many ups and downs. Some days I felt like shit, some days I felt okay. I never knew when I woke up what the day had in store for me, but I had the mental tools to keep me above the line.

At the point where I had lost thirty-five pounds and was emotionally and physically drained, I reached out for help from my coaches, especially Fran, on a regular basis. They reinforced the lessons I had learned just months before and they were able to put me on the right road once again, mentally and physically. It was my first experience seeing that even as a trained coach, I still needed input from others. This has been one of my secret keys to maintaining a positive mindset. Reaching out for help from others when I need it is a tool I use to this day.

ALONG THE SAME PATH

It's funny to look back now and realize that Lisa and I were in similar programs at the same time but in different locations. When we crossed paths here in Naples, we had not only similar cancer experiences, but we shared a language and a way of interpreting life that made us uniquely compatible. We talked for many hours about our cancer journeys and how they transformed us for the better. Because of our similar mindsets, we were able to see how together we could impact the cancer community with this positive message.

There is hope. Cancer doesn't define you, cancer is just a part of your story. Guard your mind and make it work for you, not against you. Reach out to people who can help you on dark days and know that you are not alone. Stop by our Shine Beyond Cancer Facebook page for a daily dose of positivity and leave a comment and introduce yourself. We'd love to be there to coach you today.

LISA'S MINDSET TRANSFORMATION

ROCKY BEGINNINGS

I believe we are all products of our environment but we don't have to be a victim of our environment. My childhood was no fairy tale, though from an outside perspective it may have looked that way. In stark contrast, behind closed doors, the atmosphere was volatile, full of addiction and shrouded in secrecy. "What happens in this house, stays in this house" was a family rule.

The first time I ran away from home I was four years old. I packed my Barbie suitcase and called my grandmother to come to get me. Without hesitation, she did. I would learn early on that she was my superhero. The truth is, I learned early in my life how to survive in unstable environments.

Although my family was well known in town, we weren't the Cleavers. I was exposed to addiction and high conflict situations regularly, and from this confusion and pain, I developed the art of detachment as a vital coping mechanism. I tried to avoid what was happening around me, and I didn't allow myself to feel the negative emotions of anger, sadness or insecurity. I would not allow myself to be that vulnerable. I became a "glass half full" type of girl...it felt better.

Because I had to do most things for myself and take care of my two younger brothers, I essentially lost that carefree childhood feeling and became very independent early on. These were the years I developed some debilitating limiting beliefs that I was not good enough, that it was not okay to show weakness and that if I was perfect I would be loved. On the flip side, I also developed the skills of focusing on the solutions instead of the problem. I learned resiliency and the art of setting goals.

I knew that as soon as I could, I needed to get out of the toxic environment called "home" and I planned accordingly. At the ripe old age of seventeen, I packed my bags and left for college. I spent most of my college days attending class, studying in the library and working. I didn't allow a lot of time to work on relationships. My goal was to finish and move on to the next goal. My family relationships would remain a constant struggle throughout these years.

ADULTING

I believe we are all products of our environment but we don't have to be a victim of our environment.

Although my solid emotional skills in detachment helped in difficult situations, I was never fully engaged in any of my personal relationships because I didn't allow myself to feel or express my emotions. In addition to coping with life through detachment, I also became a perfectionist. My mantra was that nothing was ever good enough. I was always striving to be the best, and that became an exhausting pattern for me because I was endlessly filling my time with work and projects. And sometimes we can't see in ourselves what is so obvious to others.

I was the perfect straight-A student in school and the best employee anyone could hire. I was an overachiever, and everything I did had to be better than everyone else's. No one could compete with my work ethic or determination. I continued to push myself harder, always striving for perfection but not allowing anyone to get close enough to see that I was really struggling with the belief that I was not good enough. Being perfect was my perfect addiction and my mask to cover up all the insecurities I carried with me from childhood.

> The definition of *mind* is "the element of a person that enables them to be aware of the world and their experiences, to think, and to feel; the faculty of consciousness and thought."

Being surrounded by addicted people in my early years and having moved on to adulthood, I had pride in never having become "one of them." I didn't realize that perfectionism is also a form of addiction, and it's a seemingly noble vice many people choose to hide from themselves. Prior to my diagnosis, I thought life was pretty great but for years I had this empty feeling—you know, the one when you are alone, in the dark, with just you and your thoughts.

PERSONAL GROWTH

I always say that my glass is half full, and even when the world is crumbling around me I focus on the solutions and try to remain positive. However, I hit a point in my life where detachment was no longer working for me. I looked around at the life that I had created, and I realized I had no emotions about anything except the pure joy I felt when I was with my daughters. What was wrong with me?

In August 2010, a friend introduced me to a personal growth course. I decided to sign up as a favor to her with no intention of actually participating for my own benefit. I didn't know I needed personal growth because I was living with the mask of perfection.

> **Without the weakness I felt, I would not have known the depth of my strength. Without the fear I felt, I would not have known how much courage I am capable of. And without the ugliness of this disease, I may never have known how full of grace I am.**

Much to my surprise, this course was the biggest gift anyone had ever given me. During that first three-day course, I listened and learned, and then I began to participate and engage and then I started to remember who I really was. It changed my life and my outlook in such an amazing way.

We did role playing and acted out things we needed to deal with. I started to figure out what was no longer serving me, and I was able to begin releasing some of the limiting beliefs I had been carrying with me for years. I learned that I was a powerful, loving, deserving leader. There had been times in my life where I would sabotage myself because I didn't feel worthy enough.

This personal growth experience took me out of my comfort zone and forced me to deal with my past, take a risk to grow up emotionally and change my ways of being. I continued on with the follow-up courses for the next several months. It is definitely in the top five best things I have ever done in my life.

CANCER AND THE GIFT

The definition of mind is "the element of a person that enables them to be aware of the world and their experiences, to think, and to feel; the faculty of consciousness and thought." We have approximately 70,000 thoughts per day and yet only about five percent of those are conscious thoughts—thoughts that we are actually aware of.

The personal growth courses that I devoured prior to the breast cancer diagnosis certainly helped me to create a vision for my life and to define more clearly who and what I wanted to be in this life. They made me vitally aware of my thoughts. I had also learned the art of responsibility and how this tool can erase a victim mentality. I am so grateful that I was able to use these tools to pull myself forward to fight the battle that laid ahead of me with grace and dignity.

This disease has truly made me more grateful and compassionate. Today I feel truly blessed. My ability to connect from a heart space more authentically as a mother, friend, trainer, and coach has improved dramatically. I have been able to go from perfectionism to striving for excellence instead. The cancer journey allowed me to feel emotions at a very raw level. Without the weakness I felt, I would not have known the depth of my strength. Without the fear I felt, I would not have known how much courage I am capable of. And without the ugliness of this disease, I may never have known how full of grace I am.

> **I believe that the positive changes that I've been able to make will allow me to be a positive change in someone else's life.**

I believe that having a negative mindset becomes a trap that is counterproductive to healing. When I got my diagnosis I already had the tools I needed to be positive, and during treatment, I had a no negativity policy for those who were in my life. I chose to allow positivity to envelop me. I began meditation and visualization practices to help clear the clutter, create a healing vision and raise my vibration. Having a clear vision of what I wanted from life helped me get through my worst days of treatment.

When Marc and I met, it was so interesting to realize how similar our life paths had been the previous six years. We had both kicked cancer's ass and done very difficult personal growth work—he in New York and me in Florida—at almost the same time. We quickly became friends and realized that we had a message that we needed to share with the world.

Now, here we are: co-authoring a book and business partners in our project, Shine Beyond Cancer. We hope to be able to guide you through the process of trading an anxious and possibly pessimistic mindset for one of positivity and possibility. We have been able to do it and we know you can too! By changing your mind, you can change your life.

THE FUTURE

I believe that we are all here to love and be loved and everything in between that teaches us to love and be loved. As humans, we are all on a unique search for greater meaning in life and discovering what life is all about. I have always been a caretaker. It comes naturally to me. I try to use this gift to the best of my ability. My grandmother instilled in me an attitude of contribution, and that is a big part of who I am. Having cancer has given me a new path for my future.

I believe life really comes down to two things: connection and contribution. Through the process of personal growth, I now know that having a connection to the people around me is so important—more important than money, cars, success or perfectionism.

After everything I have gone through, I would never wish cancer on anyone; however, I am still grateful for the experiences I had from having breast cancer. I believe that the positive changes that I've been able to make will allow me to be a positive change in someone else's life.

I encourage you to allow yourself to connect to those around you and to the world around you. Show gratitude for what you have and make a vision for your future. Get in touch with your feelings (good and bad) and learn to express them to others, because it's feeling life that really makes it special.

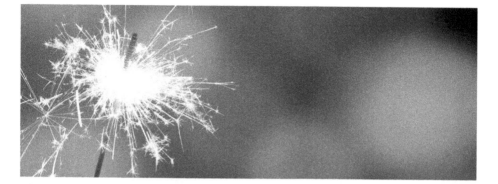

RELATIONSHIPS

At times our own light goes out and
is rekindled by a spark from another
person. Each one of us has cause to
think with deep gratitude of those who
have lighted the flame within us.

— Albert Schweitzer

MARC'S
RELATIONSHIP VALUES

MY BEGINNING

I was twenty-three when I married for the first time. My first wife gave me three beautiful daughters. But I was young and perhaps wasn't ready to be married, or be a husband. My wife was so much more mature than I was and we, unfortunately, failed to see eye to eye about many important things. In 1997, we chose to divorce. I am still and will always be grateful to her for my daughters.

Just a few short years later, I met my soulmate. Danielle and I worked on the floor together, and I knew early in the friendship that she was just right for me. Her magnetic energy brought out the best in me. It was at that point that I knew I had to be around her as much as I could. In 1999, we married and began our journey through a life that was fantastic, terrifying and, like all relationships, hard work.

Danielle and I, like any married couple, have had our ups and downs. She is the spice to my life. We enjoyed things together that I would have never done if it weren't for her. We went to Broadway shows and museums and enjoyed the nightlife of New York City. She is smart, she makes me laugh and her bubbly, friendly energy can light up a room when she walks in. But things aren't always easy.

The worst point of our marriage was when I left my career at the New York Stock Exchange. It was a tough time for us both. I felt as though I had lost the identity that I'd had for twenty-five years, and I didn't know how to react. After my heart attack and closing my business, Danielle had to shoulder the financial responsibility of our new family because my career was done. We had two young children at the time, and I couldn't cope with my sudden loss of self-worth. I was on a path of self-destruction, and I took it out on my beloved wife.

She was doing everything she could to build a new business. She was out many nights, and I was caretaking for our children. I was jealous of her new business and all the hours that it kept her from home. Instead of appreciating that she was picking up the ball I had dropped, I saw her making new friends, attending events and reading new motivational books that made me resent her success even more. I was acting like a big baby. It's a wonder that she endured my sour mood for so long. I am forever grateful that she did!

Being in that hole and trying to cope (albeit not well!) with losing something that was so important to me, I decided to go through transformational coaching in 2010. It was one of the best decisions I have ever made, for both me and Danielle. If I hadn't changed my outlook, I doubt that she and I would have made it without killing each other.

I graduated that program shortly before receiving my diagnosis in 2011. I firmly believe that absorbing what the coaching had taught me brought me to where I am now, writing this book and living my life in gratitude. Even during all of my treatments, while I was getting sicker and sicker, Danielle's and my relationship was getting better. I am appreciative of her care, love, and commitment to our relationship still to this day.

MY RELATIONSHIPS THROUGH CANCER

Although our relationship was getting stronger, it was still hard going through the cancer and treatments. At the time of my diagnosis, I had five children: Samantha was twenty-three, DJ was twenty, Brittany was eighteen, Nick was eight and Sarah was six. I have no doubt that my children were terrified during this time that they were going to lose their father. In the beginning, I felt worthless because I wasn't supporting my family financially. I was too sick to drive myself to treatment, and I was tired all the time! Danielle was there keeping our family and our finances together. On the drive to chemo and while I was getting my treatments, she was working her business, making phone calls and handling details all while still focusing on me and the things that I needed. There is no way to show her my appreciation for what she did and still does for me. She is the most exceptional woman I know!

Although Danielle and I were strong together, my relationship with my ex-wife was contentious. We argued often, mostly about money. Fortunately, during chemo, her attitude and opinion toward me changed. I think she realized that our three daughters were scared. They could lose their dad, and she was there offering them emotional support. She realized that she wanted her daughters to have their father to be there for them. So, she changed her attitude and became giving and caring, and started checking up on me and Danielle as well. My relationship with my ex-wife was probably the biggest transformation during my cancer. It was a relief that we didn't fight as often, and she was on my team on this rocky road of cancer.

It was amazing for me to see my friends and family be completely supportive and steady throughout my fight. They came to the hospital and checked on me throughout the whole process. I know some people going through cancer find that some of their friendships weren't as solid as they thought, but my friends from high school and coaching were all solid. They were there for me for whatever I needed. I felt the love flow around me and that also helped to keep the positive mindset I needed to fight the cancer.

DANIELLE AND ME POST-CANCER

When a couple goes through what we did, there are always changes. Danielle and I still have challenges, like any married couple, but we smooth them out together. Since my cancer, we have been working toward building our financial independence once again. We decided to leave New Jersey and move to Florida just eighteen months after my stem cell transplant. I found the peace I needed for myself, and our family has adjusted to year-round sunny weather and living just a short bicycle ride from the beach. I honestly don't know how I endured so many winters! We have enjoyed a change of scenery, and my need to recover and relax has been fulfilled.

> **Instead of being a self-centered businessman, I am now a heart-centered entrepreneur.**

After moving to Florida, I realized I had changed a great deal. No longer was I the driven, money-hungry businessman that I had been in New York. I began to wonder if being that businessman was what had made me sick. I know my cancer was caused from volunteering in the pit during 9/11 but did my lifestyle exacerbate that? I realized that I no longer wanted to live pedal to the metal, eight hours a day, every day of the week. It has been an adjustment for everyone. Danielle tries to understand this change in me, but sometimes she doesn't.

It's hard to explain how cancer has changed who I am and how it has rearranged my values and ideals. Instead of being a self-centered businessman, I am now a heart-centered entrepreneur. Instead of running myself into the ground, I now take time to relax and enjoy life. Today I see the value in having balance. Having a successful business and being present for my family is a well-deserved change and one that Danielle and I are both learning to embrace.

LOOKING TO THE FUTURE

Today, Danielle and I understand each other. We are different people with different talents and skills, and we realize that open communication is essential. We have a unique partnership and have grown so much together. We work a business together, we work out together, we walk the beach together and enjoy our weekly date nights. I'm so grateful to have her by my side no matter what. Sometimes she might run and I might walk but we are still going to get there in the end, together. That's a beautiful place to be with someone who means so much to you.

RELATIONSHIP ADVICE

If you are having to reinvent your relationships during and after cancer, realize that it's totally normal. Don't hold anything back. Tell your partner or family how you feel. Be willing to tell them what you need. It's liberating to just get it out. Sometimes it may not be what the other person wants to hear, but having a mature conversation and listening to each other can make things work out. There can always be a middle ground. Be grateful for the people you have around you and show them that their love is reciprocated. Slow down and enjoy all the moments you possibly can and be grateful for them.

> **Tell your partner or family how you feel. Be willing to tell them what you need. It's liberating to just get it out.**

LISA'S RELATIONSHIP VALUES

FAMILY DYNAMICS

My family life was rather complicated. My parents came from vastly different backgrounds. My mother was a farm girl from rural Allen County, Ohio. My father came from the city and was part of the country club scene.

On top of that, I grew up in an emotionally charged and toxic environment. As a child, I taught myself relationship skills to keep myself sane in the midst of uncertainty and trauma. What worked best was to just detach emotionally. This one strategy helped me to survive my home environment.

I learned to show no emotion whatsoever. I rarely dealt with any negative emotions like fear, anger or sadness. I just put on a happy face and tried to be as non-confrontational as possible. I avoided conflicts and that served me well throughout my childhood. This even helped throughout college, but when I became an adult I realized I needed to change. These well-rehearsed and ingrained survival tactics weren't working anymore, but I had never learned anything else.

Throughout childhood, I was an enabler and caretaker for those around me. I am an empath. I am sensitive to the energy and emotion of the people around me. It got more intense as I reached adulthood. My empathic nature attracts a certain personality type, and a lot of the time those

> I knew the road ahead was going to be difficult and wrought with change, but with the help of my friends and family, I knew I could get through it.

people are rather narcissistic. This relationship normally works, the narcissist is getting all the attention they need and the empath is the nurturer until something happens that causes the dynamic to shift 180 degrees.

For me, this was the dynamic of my marriage and it worked well for us both until it didn't. In a three-year period, I lost my father, my thirty-six-year-old brother and my grandmother, who was my role model. My survival instinct to detach kicked into high gear. I would not grieve or show anger (for years). I was resentful toward my husband, at the time, but would not create conflict. His inability to take care of me emotionally, and my unwillingness to let him, made our marriage difficult and frustrating. I buried my thoughts and feelings, put a smile on my face, and kept the facade of my perfect little life with my perfect kids and my perfect job.

MAKING CHANGES

It wasn't until 2004 that I realized how unhappy I was. I remember looking in the mirror one day and I said out loud, "I have no idea who you are." I was in my thirties and had completely lost myself. I didn't even know who I wanted to be. So, I started working to figure it out.

I left my marriage and moved to Florida with my daughters. I bought every self-help book I could find and devoured them. I started therapy but that didn't last long. I didn't want to talk about my marriage or my past. I knew that I needed to grieve the losses I had endured, but I had no idea how to do that. When I entered that therapist's office, I told her what we were going to talk about and what we weren't. That didn't work out at all because that's not how therapy works. But that was the first time I had been willing to dig deeper into myself or put any effort into finding out who I was. It was a step in the right direction.

It was then that I realized that before I could deal with the past, I needed to figure me out first. I couldn't even think of creating a healthy, positive relationship with anyone else until I had one with myself. My separation and subsequent divorce really spurred me into lots of personal growth. After putting in the work on myself, I was finally able to deal with all the emotions I had suppressed over the years and allow myself to feel things. I learned the healthy way to grieve my losses and celebrate my successes.

DEALING WITH CANCER

When I was told by the doctor that I had breast cancer, I didn't hear anything he said after he told me. When I got to my car, I screamed at the top of my lungs, *"Are you fucking kidding me?"* and I was angry! Because of my prior experience with personal growth, I was able to express that and feel that anger to its fullest. I knew the road ahead was going to be difficult and fraught with change, but with the help of my friends and family, I knew I could get through it.

People come into your life for a reason, a season or a lifetime. While some were exiting my life, there were so many more amazing people stepping into my life.

My most important relationships are with my daughters. I knew throughout treatment that I would have to be strong for them. They were my motivation; my inspiration to fight. I was warned that I would have good days and bad days. But I had the tools I needed to deal with the emotional toll cancer was going to put on me. Finally, I was able to allow myself to feel the emotions and, on bad days, we cried; on good days, we laughed. I have no doubt that my girls were afraid. My daughters were fifteen and eighteen years old at the time and were facing the possibility of losing their mother. I can't even begin to imagine what that felt like for them, but I knew through the whole thing that I was going to have to be strong, positive and open with my daughters as much as possible. My relationship with them was my strength throughout cancer and has been a highlight of my life, but not all relationships survive cancer.

One of the biggest shifts I experienced was actually the loss of relationships. I lost three of my closest friends during my battle. I told everyone in my circle that there was a "No Negativity Policy" in full effect. I needed to have a very positive vibe around me. I needed to focus on my energy and my healing. I understand that it is difficult for loved ones to endure watching someone fight for their life. They don't know what to do for you or what to say. What they don't realize is that much of the time, they don't need to do or say anything and just be there. So I chose to have some difficult conversations and create some distance between me and anyone who was dumping negative energy into my space. At the time, I was actually more relieved than upset because finally, it was no longer about them. They didn't understand how to be supportive.

> On my bathroom mirror, I have my mantra written in red Sharpie marker that reads, "I am willing to love myself exactly as I am."

People come into your life for a reason, a season or a lifetime. While some were exiting my life, there were so many more amazing people stepping into my life. My two best friends, Louise and Molly, were in the trenches with me through it all. Their unwavering support for me and my girls, still to this day, makes my heart full. Clients who I had just started working with before my diagnosis showed up at chemo with green smoothies, searched for alternative treatments and hung in there with me. One friend, Nikki, who I had just recently met through a mutual friend, lived in Michigan and flew back down to Florida to go to one of my chemo treatments with me. I met a total stranger in the grocery store right before Thanksgiving who asked if I was battling cancer and requested my address just to send me a care package. It was the most uplifting experience. It was an amazing feeling, and I realized that there are good humans in the world.

You never know who will be on your path. Sometimes people in your life need to step off the path for their own growth as well as yours. But you should always remain open to the people who want to walk with you, support you and love you.

> **The most important relationship to cultivate is the one in the mirror. When you are willing to love yourself, when you know that you are good enough and when you feel worthy, you are able to love and be loved.**

BOUNDARIES

Everyone deals with cancer differently. I knew I needed to have positivity and healthy relationships around me. So, I came up with a few boundaries for myself that I felt would help me and those around me get through cancer and the treatments.

The first was the No Negativity Policy. The second was the 24-Hour Rule. Each time there was a new test, new result, another procedure, I wanted 24 hours to allow myself space to wrap my head around it before others gave me their opinions. It was kind of a personal quarantine that allowed me to process not only the information but also the emotions. The third was allowing myself to ask for help. Asking for help from those who love and care about you allows them to contribute and allows you to receive their joy.

Cancer taught me how to receive. It was always hard for me to ask for anything from anyone. I was always the one who was giving, doing things for others. I was the strong one who didn't need help. I learned through personal growth that by not allowing others to give to you, that you are actually taking away from them.

And the fourth, you know that song by Frank Sinatra, *My Way?* Yep, this was my journey, my lesson, my blessing and I was doing it MY way. I encourage you to do the same.

LOVE "YOU"!

Cancer changes your perception on a lot of things. It made me realize that I had to stand up for myself. On my bathroom mirror, I have my mantra written in red Sharpie marker that reads, "I am willing to love myself exactly as I am." I read it every day; sometimes more than once. It reminds me that I don't have to be perfect. I think that when you are in a good place with yourself, that you attract the people who are supposed to be in your life. For me, eighteen years ago, I never would have imagined myself writing a book and being open and vulnerable to anyone. I was unwilling to allow that because it left me open to being hurt. The personal growth I went through changed that perception.

My personal growth is something that I still work on. I work every day at letting go of old behaviors, limiting beliefs and guarding my emotions. Allowing myself to be emotionally vulnerable to others is difficult, but I do it anyway. I'm not perfect, but I believe that we are an ongoing masterpiece. Everything that comes our way teaches us something new about ourselves and allows us to create more valuable relationships. We offer our personal growth work in more detail on our website. You will find bonus tools at www.shinebeyondcancer.com/toolbox.

The most important relationship to cultivate is the one in the mirror. When you are willing to love yourself, when you know that you are good enough and when you feel worthy, you are able to love and be loved.

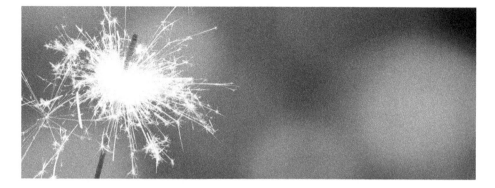

CAREER

I've missed more than 9,000 shots in my career. I've lost almost 300 games. 26 times, I've been trusted to take the game winning shot and missed. I've failed over and over and over again in my life. And that is why I succeed.

— *Michael Jordan*

MARC'S CAREER PATH

WHEN I GROW UP

I always knew I wanted to follow in my father's footsteps and be a part of the financial industry when I reached adulthood. I grew up listening to his stories about being a New York Stock Exchange broker. We often sat around the kitchen table and I would listen intently as he shared the action and buzz about his busy day. I had the opportunity, on a few occasions, to visit him on the floor while he worked and the adrenaline was palpable.

Throughout high school, I played football and wanted to continue to play in college. Being a die-hard athlete, I often let sports take over the time I should have been using for my studies. The bad news was that after eighteen months of paying for my college education, with little scholastic results to show for it, my dad pulled the plug. While I was disappointed, I understood that college may not be for me so I thought through my next steps and the decision seemed obvious. I started my career at the New York Stock Exchange at the ripe old age of twenty.

At that time, new brokers didn't really need an interview; instead, they needed someone already on the floor to get them in the door and I had that with my father. He knew so many people and was able to quickly get me a placement with a firm. So, within months, there I was moving up the ranks quickly and soon started making a lot of money.

While my friends, who at the time were juniors and seniors in college, were hitting the books, I was working and bringing home decent paychecks on Fridays. On weekends, I would hang out with my friends and, more often than not, pay for whatever we wanted to do. After all, I was a working man and they were just students.

But my lack of maturity showed when I often had to borrow money from my dad come Monday morning to get to work and make it through the week until Friday's payday. I'm sure he was less than thrilled at me for blowing my check every weekend, but he still helped me out.

STARTING WORK

My career quickly flourished and I was good at what I did. It was 1983, and the country was coming out of the recession and the economy was picking up. Business was good. I went from firm to firm until I finally found one that felt like home. I married and had three beautiful daughters during this time and continued to make good money doing what I enjoyed.

But success in business does not always result in success in life. My marriage was crumbling, and I was ready for a change. My ex-wife and I knew that what we had was not going to get better, and although my daughters were young, I was confident I could still be a great father to them. So we decided to end our marriage.

Within a few years, I divorced my first wife and once again switched to a different firm. It was at Salomon Brothers that I met Danielle. We worked in close proximity on the floor, and her energy was magnetic. My career was thriving and my reputation was growing. So in 1996, when Salomon Brothers announced a merger with Smith-Barney, I took a big risk and started an independent business on the New York Stock Exchange in January of 1997.

Starting off with no customer base at all, I used my long-standing relationships to quickly bring in business. Within the first month, I turned a sizeable profit. By May of 1997, I had more business than I could ever imagine, so I hired my friend David Fox, who I knew and trusted since I was ten years old, to join our business.

Between 1999 and 2002, life was on the upswing; things exploded on the floor for us. We were making phenomenal money, I had Danielle and Fox by my side, and I had the privilege of working alongside eight other employees whom I deeply cared for. We were a team, and the sky was the limit. My business was successful beyond even my wildest dreams. I was so happy and grateful with the path my life was on.

BIG CHANGES AHEAD

Although I was an independent businessman running a money-making firm, I lacked the foresight to see the changes that were coming with the onslaught of computers and technology. Within a short period of time, computers started taking over trading. This sudden switch to technology blindsided me and unfortunately, I didn't react quickly enough to adjust to the changes. With eight employees' salaries, payroll taxes and rent, our expenses were exorbitant. I had to make at least $100,000 a month just to cover our overhead! Revenue was dipping, expenses were up and I was desperately trying to keep it all together. It wasn't long before my body couldn't take the stress anymore and I had a heart attack.

A DIFFERENT OUTLOOK

I was hospitalized with a stress-related heart attack on August 1, 2006. After three months of recuperation, I came back to the floor with every intention of picking up where I left off. When I finally returned, I realized very quickly that my career as a floor broker was over. The open outcry system of the New York Stock Exchange that had been in place for 200 years was slowly being wiped out by the impersonal and instantaneous trading that computers offered. The expertise that I had wasn't valued as much as the speed of execution. The Christmas of 2006 was the hardest time for me. I made a decision to close my business. Leaving the floor behind, I knew in the coming year I had to reinvent myself.

The fact that I was no longer a broker was something that I had a hard time coming to terms with and still do. When your identity and your social life revolves around a twenty-five-year career, finding something else is extremely difficult. I was depressed and disillusioned. Where else could I go that would give me the same adrenaline? Where else could I use the unique skills I had developed as a floor broker to make as much money as I was used to making? Where else could I be my own boss and have fun with my friends every day? The outlook seemed bleak.

Losing that part of my identity turned out to be more challenging than I had ever imagined. I was a wreck! Knowing I had to try to find work and make money, I jumped to different trading desks and became the person I didn't like when I was on the floor. I was the guy giving orders and telling people what to do. That option just didn't work for the type of person I am, so I left.

Through a slew of job changes and different positions, I never found a place that felt like home. For the five years following my heart attack, I was struggling with my emotions, my health, and my mental state. It was a chaotic and frustrating point in my life that didn't seem to have an end in sight.

ADJUSTING TO MY DIAGNOSIS

There are so many things that, I believe, contributed to my cancer. For sure it came from my time in the toxic environment in the pit while volunteering during 9/11. To this day I can vividly remember the fires burning, the smoke, the ash, the dust and the smell of burnt metal. You could just smell disaster. The commotion of thousands of people doing whatever they could to help all in organized chaos. Trying to find survivors was the main goal in those first forty-eight hours. Of all the things that Danielle and I experienced in the pit one thing really stands out. You would hear the Fire Chief on the bullhorn ask for silence when the search dogs started barking and stopped at an area. You could sense the prayers and hope of thousands of us as they dug and cut beams away to see if there was anyone alive. Unfortunately, during those first few days, we were unable to find any survivors.

Couple all of that with the stress and negative energy I was dealing with on a daily basis inside and out. I went from a high adrenaline job on the floor, to a low energy environment for the five years following my heart attack. All of these things contributed to my bad vibes and poor mental state along with feeling sick all the time for no apparent reason. I was angry and frustrated and desperately needed a positive change.

I was not in a good place and was getting sicker and sicker from an accidental fall I had while walking down the icy stairway to my gym, which was misdiagnosed as Epstein-Barr mono and was later diagnosed as stage 4 Hodgkin's lymphoma. So not only was I lost in my career, but I was also losing my health. At my darkest moment, a light started to shine through.

My health began to get better when Danielle found a nutritional program that turned things around. It helped me put on weight, and my mind began to clear. I started to feel an inner peace as my body was responding to the dense superfood regimen we had been introduced to through a friend.

At this point, Danielle and I realized that there was a virtual franchise business possibility with this nutritional product line. It is a US-based company that is family-owned, and you could operate your franchise online. All the products ship directly to your customers from their warehouse, and customer support was handled by the company too. We couldn't believe our eyes! Was this my next career move? Operating an online franchise business helping people with the nutrition that was helping me so much? This was a product I believed in then and still do today, so why would it not work for others? Wasn't it my responsibility to pay it forward? My wheels started turning. I believe in what this company did for me, so Danielle and I decided to go into business together to give others the gift of health.

A NEW BUSINESS PLAN

Although I was still struggling to find my identity and a good way to make money, this seemed to be a viable opportunity to meet these needs and try something totally different. We didn't feel we had anything to lose because it had such a low barrier of entry. For under $1,000, we had our website up and running and were ready to start marketing it to our friends and family. Fortunately, Danielle and I both possess an entrepreneurial mindset, and with an understanding of how to build our client base to maximize our revenues, we decided to go full force.

Danielle and I are also both driven for success. At this point in my life, however, Danielle had more drive than I did. After a heart attack and cancer, I needed a little bit of time to not be the crazy obsessed man I had been when I was a floor broker. I feel like being that person had contributed to my sickness. So I became the sidekick to my wife and her fast-paced persona. We worked hard to be successful in our new venture and fortunately, our dream came to fruition.

In just over five years, Danielle and I became the 253rd representatives to make a million dollars cumulatively in our company. For us, it was an honor to have received that recognition and we know that the number isn't what is important. It's what the number represents. It means that we have helped over 27,000 people change their health for the better. We are blessed to have been successful in this business and to have gone through the financial and life changes that we did.

REVELATIONS

After struggling with reinvention and feeling like I had lost my identity, I realized that life is full of opportunities and ups and downs. As cliche as it sounds, life is a roller coaster. It is not easy, and it rarely ever goes the way you planned it to. With this insight and foresight, I was looking for the next step and the next new challenge, and that is precisely when I met Lisa. We had both survived stage four cancer and had both gone through the same coaching program, in different states, at about the same time. Soon our vision was born and we began Shine Beyond Cancer.

Danielle and I have always wanted an opportunity that puts us in charge of our destiny, and the nutrition business has given us just that. Now I feel it's time to work more specifically with people who have been touched by cancer, like me, and help them in every area to create a life beyond cancer that surpasses their wildest dreams. Lisa's story is similar to mine, and she wants the same thing too. It's exciting to know that I can create a business helping people reinvent themselves and change their destiny even while going through cancer.

> **As cliche as it sounds, life is a roller coaster. It is not easy, and it rarely ever goes the way you planned it to.**

This is my drive. I found it again, and I understand that I can't just sit and be content where I am. After this battle, I know there is still more. More for me to do, earn, contribute and experience—all of it. Danielle and I are on the same page with that.

THINGS CAN CHANGE

You can change careers; you are not stuck where you are right now. If you aren't fulfilled with what you're currently doing, start by looking at your options and making a list of what you are naturally good at and what you enjoy. To be sure, making a change requires some faith and a tolerance for a season of uncertainty. But it is all worth it.

> **You are the captain of your vessel, and you can get what you want if you are willing to dream and take some action.**

Making a change is ultimately a choice, and when you face cancer you understand in a way many don't that life is precious and it's crucial to spend every minute doing something you love and helping others in the process.

Lisa and I want to inspire and encourage you to try something else if you are feeling stuck in your career. Start a side hustle. Create time for a hobby that could grow into an income stream. Look online at virtual franchises and talk with friends who have successfully changed careers. There are so many more opportunities out there than there used to be. Remember that you get to choose your path in all aspects of your life; your career is one of those areas.

You are the captain of your vessel, and you can get what you want if you are willing to dream and take some action. Lisa and I are here to be the wind beneath your wings to inspire you to do that.

LISA'S CAREER PATH

A SALES STAR IS BORN

Sales and hospitality were ingrained in me from childhood. Like most girls of a young age, I was a Girl Scout. My first taste of success in sales was Girl Scout cookies. Yep, I was top salesgirl! I definitely got this talent from my father. Growing up, I also had an artistic, creative side, which was a gift from my Dad as well.

When I went to college at the University of Cincinnati, I enrolled as a business major, which seemed natural but the second quarter I switched directions and decided to major in art. My father soon pointed out that being an artist wasn't going to pay the bills, so I changed my major back to business and marketing. My goal was to have a corner office with a view in a high-rise in Manhattan on Madison Avenue selling everything to everyone.

BECOMING THE CAREER WOMAN

After graduation, I entered the hospitality industry (which was a family tradition) and began working at a resort in Florida. It was my first hotel job. I was young and motivated so I was willing to move around a lot. I wanted to see the world (or run away from the reality of my family and feelings). My next hotel job would take me to the west coast, Southern California.

I eventually found my hospitality home (and my future husband) with Hyatt Hotels. In 1989, my future husband and I landed in New Orleans. He was transferred there with Hyatt and I followed. I went to work for the New Orleans Convention Bureau as a National Accounts Salesperson. Seriously, my job was to showcase the best of New Orleans to convention planners. It was such a fun job! It was my first "real" sales job. I traveled a lot for trade shows. I was energized by the pursuit of the next sale. I was a born saleswoman, I was good at my job and loved it.

My husband and I married in 1991 and threw a traditional New Orleans wedding. We would live in New Orleans for three more years.

In 1994, seven months pregnant with our first daughter, Veronica, we were transferred to Columbus, Ohio. I had the opportunity to be a stay-at-home mom, which is certainly a full-time job, but I missed the excitement of my professional life. I needed to figure out a way to have both.

> I wasn't sure I would be able to pull off having two adorable little girls at home and still feed my professional desire. I would have to reinvent myself again.

While in Columbus, I contacted the visitor's bureau and sent them a proposal that would allow me to work from home but still maintain my connection to the hospitality world. We stayed in Columbus for only a year.

Next stop, Washington, DC. I loved living in DC and contacted my former boss in New Orleans because the New Orleans Convention Bureau had a DC office. I still wanted to be home with my now one-year-old bundle of joy, but I couldn't wait to start making those sales calls.

New Orleans gladly took me back but wanted me in the DC office five days a week. My father used to say I could sell ice to Eskimos, but what I really needed was to sell a flex-time work option to New Orleans. They bought! I would work for New Orleans while at home for half the week and then the other half of the week I would be in the office. This turned out to be a dream. I was still able to witness Veronica hitting those toddler milestones, and shortly thereafter we prepared for another bundle of joy. Olivia was on her way.

Hyatt loved to move us while I was pregnant. Next stop, Dearborn, Michigan and in the middle of winter in 1998...ugh! I wasn't sure I would be able to pull off having two adorable little girls at home and still feed my professional desire. I would have to reinvent myself again. Shortly after arriving in Dearborn, I met the mayor of Dearborn, a perk of having the hotel connection. I became his campaign and fundraising manager. That was a full-time job, but it was perfect for me as I could work from home or bring my children with me. Life was good! I truly had the best of both worlds.

Life loves to throw curveballs.

After the mayor's campaign was over, he loaned me out to a US senator and I ran a national campaign, which was a lot of fun. Throughout the campaign, I was still responsible for the mayor's fundraisers, projects and initiatives. I wasn't an employee of the city or state, but I was working on the mayor's PR stuff.

I always loved moving to a new city and rediscovering myself again and again. It's difficult for me to imagine myself in an office for eight hours a day, so all the moves and reinvention really satisfied my adventurous and creative side. I had full flexibility with all my jobs to work, raise my girls and focus on my health and exercise.

After all the campaigns were finished, I had a lot more free time. I chose another new career path...real estate. It wasn't long after passing the state exam that I acquired my first listing and also procured the buyer for that listing. I felt like I had found my niche, sales and making people's dreams come true! Very quickly, I rose to number three in a large real estate company.

I was still able to spend ample amounts of time with my kids, and they often attended open houses on Sundays with me. I was able to arrange my schedule around my family's schedule and although I was busy it was never an excuse to not be there for my girls. I was assisting in campaigns, balancing my real estate career and participating as PTO president. I didn't feel overworked or stressed out about all the directions I was running; instead, I felt full satisfaction with my life and its path.

A TIME FOR CHANGE

Life loves to throw curveballs. While living in Michigan, after the deaths of my father, grandmother, and brother in a three-year period, I made a very difficult decision to leave my marriage, and the girls and I moved to Florida. I got a Florida real estate license and shortly after that decided to get my broker's license as well. I realized quickly that the Naples real estate market was completely different from Dearborn. Helping people find their second or third home didn't have the same satisfaction for me as when I was helping someone find their dream home for their family.

No longer did I enjoy my job, so I changed angles. I started working for a commercial developer and began developing whole communities. The pressure of the major life changes I had recently made in my life and career path started surfacing. My girls and I were in a new city with virtually no friends for support, and I was under enormous amounts of stress. I felt like I was going through it all alone: being a single parent, working in a new career, unraveling my past, and dealing with difficult emotions.

This was where the real personal growth would begin. The time to reinvent myself once again had arrived—but this time it was different. This time, it would be about purpose and passion. I was willing to do a lot of internal work. It wasn't all smooth sailing, and truth be told there were lots of trials and errors for a period of six years.

DISCOVERING MY PURPOSE

In 2010, I really began to focus on myself and the vision I had for my life. This was the beginning of my obsession with Power Plate and personal training.

In 2012, the year before my cancer diagnosis, I decided that opening a Power Plate studio was what I really wanted to do. I wanted to empower and enhance the lives of others through personal training and coaching. I started with a business plan, got the training that I needed to bring awareness to people about the benefits of whole body vibration.

In February 2013, I opened my business from scratch and began growing my clientele. I had a vision and the drive for success, and I was working hard to get there. When I was diagnosed with cancer, within the first few months of my studio opening, I had about thirty clients. Throughout my diagnosis and treatment, I never missed a day of training. I was able to schedule clients around my treatment appointments, and that is the beauty of having my own business. It was important to me not to lose my dream, just because the road ahead was going through some construction.

The time to reinvent myself once again had arrived—but this time it was different. This time, it would be about purpose and passion.

I shared studio space with my original Power Plate trainer. I put the dream of having my own studio on hold during my treatments because the treatments themselves felt like a full-time job. After I finished all the treatments, my drive for my own studio went into high gear. I used a non-profit agency called SCORE and they helped me build my business plan.

I never doubted that I was going to have a studio. It makes me laugh looking back at that first meeting with the SCORE mentor to discuss my ideas for the business plan. I had just finished cancer treatment, I was bald, I was pretty much broke from paying for the treatments and I had no investor. The guy must have thought I was crazy, but there was nothing that was going to stop me from opening this studio and fulfilling my dream.

> When I got my diagnosis, I knew I had to fight all the way through treatment and beyond. I am grateful that my cancer experience has given me even more passion for helping others, for adding another dimension to my career and for the pure joy of living a healthy, vibrant life.

Five years have gone by since that meeting, and I have a thriving wellness studio. I have multiple streams of income as well. For some, maybe the studio would have been enough but I have always been a determined woman. I became a distributor for BEMER, the medical device that changed my life, and I am currently in the top one percent of the company in the US.

THOUGHTS AND CHANGE

When I got my diagnosis, I knew I had to fight all the way through treatment and beyond. I am grateful that my cancer experience has given me even more passion for helping others, for adding another dimension to my career and for the pure joy of living a healthy, vibrant life. Cancer has made me feel invincible.

Yes, there were times when I felt exhausted and sick and worn out, but I knew I had a vision for myself, for my girls and for my clients, so I just kept going. I was cancer broke and yet I still managed to build my dream career. And I'm still building!

Don't give up! You may have to work your ass off to get to where you want to be. I know that I did. But is it really work if you are creating an opportunity for yourself from your heart? Give yourself the chance to look at all areas in your life from a different perspective, the cancer perspective. You can reinvent your career, and now is the perfect time to do it. Shine on!

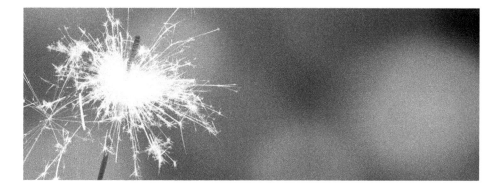

FINANCES

Fortune sides with him who dares.

– Virgil

MARC'S FINANCIAL ROLLER COASTER

WHAT TO FOCUS ON

My grandfather passed suddenly from a brain tumor when my father was just thirteen and that, I believe, changed my father's outlook on life and money. Losing his father the way he did, my dad realized that life is fragile and it can end abruptly. My parents have always been givers. They were relatively free-flowing when it came to money. We went away on vacations and out to dinner. My parents enjoyed taking us on different experiences. It was a lesson my father instilled in me as well. Because of this outlook, he has lived a happy and abundant life and has not hoarded his money for a rainy day. He taught me to live and enjoy every single day.

I took these lessons into my young adult years. My business was successful, and it was easy to be relaxed about money. I didn't worry, and I had more than any kid from Brooklyn could have dreamed. Once computerization came along and I closed my business, the financial strain started taking a toll. How would I bring in enough money to support my kids? I felt like the rug was pulled out from under me.

After my heart attack, I realized that I could no longer handle the stresses that came with being a high-level broker, so I began working in sales, trading for different firms around New York. I was unhappy, and my boss and I mutually came to the decision that this wasn't the best fit for me.

Because I was laid off, I didn't have any health insurance and I was scared of what that meant.

Not only was my health declining, but my bank account had been dissolved also. Although my wife was working and making money for our household at the time, she wasn't making enough for the COBRA payments, which were $1,400 a month, so I let my insurance go. To add insult to injury, shortly after I was let go was when I was diagnosed with cancer. It was terrifying to realize that when I got my diagnosis, I had no insurance to help pay for my treatments. I didn't know what to do next, but I held on to my abundant mindset and knew that we would get through it somehow.

> I don't want to sound overly spiritual or crazy, but I think James Allen is right when he says, "As a man thinketh in his heart, so shall he be."

We all know that cancer treatments are expensive, but I truly had no idea how much of a financial hit we would take. Even though I was used to enjoying the finer things in life, nice restaurants, international vacations, and luxury experiences, spending money to regain my health was a whole new ball game.

It's terrifying when you are sick and the bills just keep coming, and you don't know what to do or how to get out of it. I understand that feeling and that fear. Trying to figure out how to rob Peter to pay Paul is a balancing act that is terrifying. But that is where watching your thinking really comes into play. If you think you're never going to make it, then that's what you'll create in your reality. I don't want to sound overly spiritual or crazy, but I think James Allen is right when he says, "As a man thinketh in his heart, so shall he be."

What you think about is what becomes. I really believe that having a positive and abundant mindset about finances will help your health and recovery along. It certainly proved to work for me when I was going through this awful time in my life.

You can't live with the fear that having cancer will bankrupt you. Worrying about money and how bills will get paid is a direct inhibitor to healing. So I chose my mindset going through treatment and I focused on abundance, in money, and in healing. I often had to remind myself that I am alive and I am fighting, and I had to have gratitude for that. Know that there is always a way to earn money.

THE EFFECT OF MONEY AND THE MIND

I would describe myself as a man who is proud to a fault. I am a giving, charitable person and I have a hard time receiving anything—whether it's a birthday present or even a Christmas gift. To be honest, I get a weird feeling in my stomach when someone gives me anything. I show my gratitude for the present, but I still don't like receiving things. I'm not exactly sure why I feel this way but quite simply, I do.

My Aunt Linda and my cousin Wendy know this about me, and they also love me to a fault. Little did I know they were orchestrating an amazing feat behind my back, and if I had known about what they were planning it would have been against my will. They started a charity in my name to help us secure health insurance to cover the cost of treatments. They orchestrated a fundraiser and sent marketing materials out to friends, family, and people on the New York Stock Exchange and were able to raise nearly $50,000.

It was amazing, and the feelings I had when I learned they were doing this, *for me,* were overwhelming. We were able to use the funds to purchase health insurance and proceed with treatments. Although I am not a taker or charity case and I don't like to receive things, I am so grateful for what they did and I have thanked them a billion times for it.

After beating cancer and when I started making money again, I paid every single nickel back to all the people who donated to this charity in my

> **Especially when you are going through cancer, there will be many people who want to help you and I believe that you still need to be open and grateful to receiving.**

name. I told Danielle that I couldn't live with myself until I repaid them. As a person who is a giver, it was hard for me to receive but I needed it at that time, and in the end, I truly felt better after I had paid it back.

Even though I still struggle with receiving, it was an important lesson for me. I learned that receiving is part of the cycle of giving and to stop the flow of receiving in your life is stingy and self-centered. As much as I like to give, it's good to remember that other people like to give too and I should not prevent them from doing so. Especially when you are going through cancer, there will be many people who want to help you and I believe that you still need to be open and grateful to receiving. While it was difficult for me to take all the money that was donated, I needed it at the time, so I accepted it graciously.

Remember, you are not a charity case. They are giving to you out of their generosity and their hope for your healing because they love you and want nothing more than for you to beat cancer. Please accept it. Without the gifts that I got from all those people, I don't know where I would be today. You can always make money to repay them if you feel the need to. But when you are in a situation where you need help and someone wants to assist you, accept it. If you are like me, I implore you to swallow your pride, be humble, say thank you and figure out the rest later.

LIVING TO THE FULLEST

I am cancer-free today, and it still feels amazing to say that! But I also know the other side of that is *I had cancer*. I know how fast things can change. One doctor appointment, one phone call, one minute and things as we know them can be hugely different. Since I have been cancer-free, I'm focusing on enjoying myself every single minute and enjoying my family. We love to travel and have toured through Europe and surfed in Costa Rica with all five of my kids a couple times. The joy I get to experience in seeing their smiles means the world to me. It completely outweighs all the misery of chemo and the stem cell transplant and really puts everything in perspective. Life is great and I am alive! There are always going to be highs and lows, and it's important to remember to cherish the highs and be in the right mindset during the lows. If you would like more tools for "living life to the fullest," visit www. shinebeyondcancer.com/toolbox.

Stress and anxiety caused me to have a heart attack, so I know what it can do to the body. It's not worth it to stress over money. It's all about keeping your family healthy and being able to see their smiles; being stressed out about the financial side of things is not going to help in recovering from cancer or enjoying your life. Yes, money is important, but so is having a mental state that encourages you to see the good around you. Finances are always going to be a roller coaster ride. Whether you have five dollars or five billion dollars, there will always be seasons of success and seasons of failure. It will never be one hundred percent great one hundred percent of the time. Remember, it is okay to say "I need help" because there are people out there who want to help, and you will both be better for it.

> **Remember, it is okay to say "I need help" because there are people out there who want to help, and you will both be better for it.**

LISA'S FINANCIAL ROLLER COASTER

GROWING UP

I grew up as a member of a prominent family. My father and his family owned their own businesses, lived in affluent neighborhoods and belonged to the country club. I went to a private Catholic school, played tennis and golf and was given many advantages. We went on expensive vacations and my grandparents had second homes. At a young age, I didn't realize that not everyone had these privileges.

For me, when I went to the corner store to get a snack or pick up something for my mom, I put it on a tab. Likewise, when I ordered lunch at the country club, it was added to my parents' account. From the age of fourteen, though, I have always worked and made money, but I don't think I learned to be responsible with money. As I got older and began to interact with the real world, I quickly realized that I had to change my belief system when it came to money.

> **As I got older and began to interact with the real world, I quickly realized that I had to change my belief system when it came to money.**

During college, I had a job at a bank processing payments after hours so I would have extra money to drink at the bars. Money served a purpose, although a frivolous one, and yet I still never really felt the responsibility that came with making money. I realize now that I began to adopt my mother's concepts of money. If you really want something, you must struggle to get it. Money doesn't grow on trees and there is never enough. Those negative mantras stuck with me well into adulthood.

JOBS AND MONEY

> It wasn't until I was truly open to looking at every aspect of my life, especially my finances, that I realized I had to change those limiting beliefs I had been carrying around for years.

As an adult, I had a successful career but that never seemed like enough. Often I would work late because I wanted to make sure there was enough money. Then my husband and I married and merged our two incomes. Although my husband and I were successful and made good money, I still worked hard to make sure there was enough. However, I was still quite frivolous and never really worried about spending money either.

Life progressed pretty normally for my family and me. Our family finances had increased, I was successful in real estate and my husband was doing well in his career. As was my habit, I had my hand in other sources of income as well. Then my financial life was turned upside down when my husband and I divorced.

My daughters and I moved to Florida, and I became a struggling single mom. I raised my daughters in private school and worked hard to give them everything they wanted. Their father, thank goodness, was a huge financial support for the girls. But at that time, I always felt like I was struggling to make ends meet and the stress became a heavy weight on my shoulders.

Once I started my personal growth journey, I was forced to face my long-held negative money story. My father used to say that I went to the School of Finance, where I learned to make a dollar and spend a dollar seventy-five. I'm sure my ex-husband would agree. It wasn't until I was truly open to looking at every aspect of my life, especially my finances, that I realized I had to change those limiting beliefs I

> **That was one of the biggest lessons I learned from cancer: ask for what you need.**

had been carrying around for years. To grow financially, I needed to release what I once believed and create a new money belief. I stopped spending what I didn't have, and I worked to eliminate debt.

CANCER

And just when you think you have things figured out, here comes the curveball. I had recently started my personal training business when I was diagnosed with cancer. I was self-insured because I was self-employed. I didn't have anyone paying part or all of my insurance. No matter what kind of insurance you have, cancer is still expensive.

There are tons of added expenses that come with it. People miss work because of treatment or surgery or just from feeling sick throughout. Although I never missed work due to treatment, there was still the added expense of deductibles. I was doing a lot of natural and alternative complementary care that was not covered by insurance. But thankfully I had insurance, until the insurance company decided not to pay for ANYTHING!

I received a phone call from the oncology office the day before my seventh chemo treatment, telling me that when I came in for chemo the next day I needed to bring $4,000! My insurance company had not paid a dime for any of my treatments! This phone call terrified me and certainly tested my new-found financial mindset.

You have to create a vision for what you want your money story to look like and then you have to make that vision your reality.

Although this created additional stress for me, I knew that I deserved to have treatment and that no matter what it took I was going to get those treatments. When you have cancer, it always seems like the hits just keep coming at you. When this happened with the insurance company, I strengthened my resolve and did what I had to do to raise the money for my treatments. I made it happen with the help of friends and loved ones. My friends and I had campaigns and started a GoFundMe page. Some friends even loaned me the money. I was humbled and felt the weight of my finances ease a little bit. I used this money for treatments and at this point had no insurance.

STRUGGLING AND GROWTH

I was looking at the bills for treatment and they were totaling near the $300,000 mark. Add to this that I was opening a new studio and staring at this debt, all the while still trying to raise my kids and keep myself healthy enough to work. I knew I couldn't be defeated. I just dug in a little deeper and prayed for more strength. It was overwhelming to be in this situation, but I am glad I asked for help from those around me and I'm thankful they stepped up to the plate. I am not someone who is accustomed to asking for help, but there was nowhere else for me to turn. That was one of the biggest lessons I learned from cancer: ask for what you need.

I wasn't going to let cancer define my life, so I put the medical bills on the back burner. I moved forward in building my business and opened my studio. As every entrepreneur knows, there are struggles in that first year and many tough days. There were months early on that I had to call the landlord to ask for an extension because I was juggling money. I had learned that it was okay to ask for help, and it was easier after that cancer lesson to do so. I have no doubt the landlord didn't believe I'd still be here five years later. But I had a vision for myself, my life and my kids, and there was no stopping me.

WHAT I LEARNED

My mantra now is that money is energy and you have to keep it moving and be responsible. It's important for people to look at their habits, whether overspending or hoarding it, and change that focus to the idea that money is energy. Money, like energy, can't be stagnant. It needs to flow at whatever level you are at, whether fast or slow.

Even now, I make sure that I have a safety net, but I live for today and in the moment. I want to live and enjoy the money I have, but I am also aware of how easily that can change. That's why I have multiple income streams and put money in my safety net. I focus on abundance and contribution. I pay my good fortune forward.

You have to create a vision for what you want your money story to look like and then you have to make that vision your reality. Look at negative beliefs you have about money from your past and seek out ways to release them and create a new positive financial outlook. Ask yourself what you want to do, be and have, and then create it.

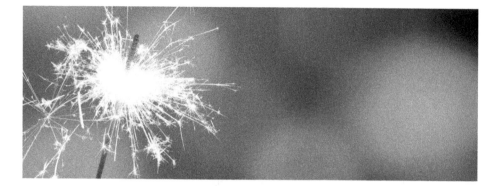

SPIRITUALITY

Faith is taking the first step, even when
you don't see the whole staircase.

– Martin Luther King, Jr.

MARC'S SPIRITUAL CONNECTION

RELIGION AND GROWTH

I grew up in a relaxed culturally Jewish home, but we never really practiced our faith with fervor like others in the Jewish community. We attended bar mitzvah services when we were invited but that was about it. I went to the obligatory religious trainings that were required of my Jewish tradition. I attended Hebrew school until I dropped out; I hated it. My parents hired a tutor to help me memorize what I needed to say, but for me, there was no real meaning behind it. I didn't feel a connection to a higher spirit, and I just went through the motions to appease my grandparents. I had a bar mitzvah when I was thirteen and that closed the end of that chapter in my Jewish upbringing.

When I reached adulthood and married, we had a Jewish ceremony and followed with the same tradition in raising our children in the faith because that was expected. My grandparents were still alive at that time, and it made them happy. So, my wife and I spent the money on the parties and did what we could to instill a basic Jewish tradition as our parents had done for us. But something wasn't working for me.

INTELLECTUALLY SPEAKING...

Despite my family's best efforts, I couldn't come to terms with spirituality or any sort of a higher power. I have always been in awe of the fact that humans have been around for millions of years and have the power to procreate. It's fascinating that animals, humans, and plants all reproduce to keep this planet thriving and intellectually, it makes sense that some higher power had to create this. It's not like building a factory that can be created and changed as necessary to keep with the plan. The development of life, as we know it, had to be flawlessly executed on the first go. But despite this awe I had of nature, I still couldn't make an emotional connection with my own spirituality.

> From the moment I got my diagnosis until I was told that I was cancer-free, I never allowed myself to be cancer's victim and that choice was important to me.

Even though I can see the good that is all around me, I had to wonder if there was a higher power that created all this greatness. If yes, then how could this higher power allow such tragedies like the Holocaust to happen? How could a higher power allow someone to crash a plane into a building and kill 3,000 people in New York City? There was no logic to it. It was hard to understand how good and evil could exist simultaneously, and why God stood by and didn't intervene to stop such awful events.

Going through cancer is one of the hardest things I have ever done. Being there to receive my treatment and seeing children go through similar treatments takes me to a very dark place. It seems so unfair and frankly, it pisses me off! These are children, innocent children; why should they have to suffer? It angered me to think that a higher power would allow it. It was hard for me to believe that some spirit in the sky would stand by to watch his children suffer from such a terrible disease. This was my problem with spirituality, and I wanted the answers to these kinds of questions.

CANCER AND NON-BELIEF

From the moment I got my diagnosis until I was told that I was cancer-free, I never allowed myself to be cancer's victim and that choice was important to me. Even though I had larger questions of God's will in world affairs and children's suffering, for some reason I never blamed God for my own cancer or thought He was punishing me. I don't believe that God gave me cancer. I knew what gave me cancer and didn't believe it to be God's plan. I know that I got cancer from being in the pit post-9/11. It was no one's fault; it was a direct result of the choices I made to stay and help at Ground Zero and remain in New York City for the six years following that tragic day. I could have left as many others did. I could have moved. But I didn't. I stayed.

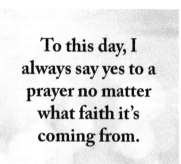

To this day, I always say yes to a prayer no matter what faith it's coming from.

After accepting that I had cancer, and knowing that I needed to learn more and remain positive, I joined Facebook groups for support. It helped me to talk to others who were going through cancer too. Often people would comment on my posts and give me their prayers. I always appreciated this and responded back respectfully even though I didn't really believe in the magic of prayers. I understood that prayer was something they could offer me that made them feel helpful. It was nice to know that people who didn't necessarily know me personally wanted to take time and pray for me. And so, I responded to them with gratitude. To this day, I always say yes to a prayer no matter what faith it's coming from.

Getting my diagnosis was the first step towards healing. When I knew what was wrong, I knew I had to fight it and I did not question whether

> I believe that gratitude is a great form of spirituality. That's the way that I want to live out the rest of my life, with gratitude.

God caused it or not. I knew I had to beat cancer for my family. I fought for them, and that's the way I thought about it. The doctors did their part. The medicines did their part. The nutrition did its part. And I'm sure the prayers of friends and family did their part.

Although I was raised Jewish, I was open to all faiths. There was a Catholic church, Saint Catherine of Siena on 68th Street, a hundred feet from New York-Presbyterian Hospital that we visited every time I went for treatments. Danielle and I would go in and say a prayer. Sometimes those prayers were twenty seconds, other times they lasted twenty minutes. The solitude and reflection helped center me. I never prayed for healing, I only prayed to see my family again. And I prayed for the spiritual comfort that it brought to me.

I had such a strong network of people to support me, and I didn't allow myself to wallow in self-pity or ask God why. I just knew that I had a family and a life that I needed to be here for, so I fought. My attitude was that I just wanted to be healthy again, and be the man that I was, or be an even better one. I am grateful I got that chance through a combination of medicine and the miraculous gift of grace. So all that combined, if you want to call it God, worked. And I won.

NEVER FIGHT ALONE

Family has always been an important part of my life. To those who are going through cancer and treatment, here is my advice. Look around you. Do you see your family and your friends? They are here for you. You are not fighting alone. You have a team around you who care deeply for you and will go to any length to help you return to perfect health. You have to fight for them...and for you. That's how it was for me. I needed to win the battle, but I knew I couldn't win by myself. It takes a village to support a cancer patient, and it takes an army to win a battle.

If you are a spiritual or religious person, add God to that equation as a positive support and healer. Be grateful for the advantages we have now when it comes to medicine. One hundred years ago, things were so much different and quite possibly your chance of recovery would not have been as optimistic as it is today. It's important not to fall into the web of asking why God gave you cancer or allowing yourself to be angry about it. This is counterproductive to healing. When you are going through a hard day, wondering if God is on your side will make that hard day worse. Remember that no matter where you are, there are resources all around you to help you to keep that positive mindset. Use them and lean on your family and friends and God if you need and keep a positive mindset with all aspects of your life, even beyond beating cancer.

GRATITUDE

I am grateful for the person who invented chemotherapy and the doctors who saved my life through the stem cell transplant. The radiation helped heal my body too. Every step I took throughout my cancer treatment saved me. A positive mindset healed my spirit and a nutritional program got me healthy again. These all played into winning my battle with cancer.

I believe that a positive mindset is crucial to incorporate with your belief in God. If you believe the path is wide open to healing, then it will be. Give gratitude to God each day. It doesn't matter if you show it by prayer and offerings to God, or by paying it forward to others who are going through a tough time.

Gratitude is huge for me. It is a spiritual practice you can use to enhance your healing. I practice gratitude in all areas of my life: my finances, my relationships, and my health. For me, there is always something to be grateful for. I am here, I beat cancer, I can see and talk to my family wherever they are and whenever I want thanks to technology. I am grateful for all that and more.

By the grace of God, my sister was a match to me and she chose to donate her stem cells. There are people out there who donate anonymously for cancer patients, and I am grateful to them as well. They help people who don't have a match available through their family. I give gratitude in every way that I can.

My advice for those who have a similar story to mine is simple. Just give gratitude to God or medicine it doesn't matter. It is what it is. There is no point in blaming God or being the victim to cancer. It's a much healthier approach to remove those negative thoughts going through the treatment process and in your life after cancer. I've said it before and I will continue to say that a positive mindset will make all the difference. Placing the blame on something or someone else gives away your power.

For me, I could have blamed Osama bin Laden and those who blew up the Twin Towers. That's what caused the dust cloud, and the dust cloud gave me cancer. But that's not the way I want my story to be written. I made the choice to stay and help the people affected. I had the free will to move away if I wanted to a place where I would have been safe, but instead, I chose to stay. We all have the free will to choose a different path. Life is all about the choices we make. That's the way I live my life: having the options to choose what I want to do and where I want to be and giving gratitude for the fact that I am here. I believe that gratitude is a great form of spirituality. That's the way that I want to live out the rest of my life, with gratitude.

LISA'S SPIRITUAL CONNECTION

CATHOLIC UPBRINGING

I was born and raised in an Irish Catholic family and attended Catholic schools. My earliest religious memory was when I received my first communion and I thought it was the best event ever! After all, my grandmother handmade my pretty new dress, we had a big party and there were presents! But I knew I didn't really understand it all. I attended daily religion classes during school, but they still didn't make sense to me. I believe Catholicism gave me a good foundation of values and taught me to treat others as I want to be treated. Throughout my younger years, I believed all the Bible stories, as most children do, but upon attending high school my views began to change.

I felt a connection to a higher power, but I no longer believed that it had to be attached to specific religious dogma.

Much to my grandmother's dismay, I stopped attending church services during high school. As always, she was understanding in that, as a teenager, I wanted to find my own path. I wouldn't attend church again until I was in my late twenties, right before my marriage. We got married in the

Catholic church and in order to do so, we had to go through Pre-Cana, a Catholic marriage prep school. I went through the motions, but there was so much that I questioned. My views of the world were different. I felt a connection to a higher power, but I no longer believed that it had to be attached to specific religious dogma.

RAISING MY FAMILY

I think as adults we follow in the footsteps of our own upbringing despite our upbringing. When my daughters were old enough to attend school, ironically enough, I enrolled them in a Catholic grade school. I wanted them to have the same foundation of values that I had, and I hadn't clearly figured out my own spirituality. We didn't take them to church on Sundays, but they received their sacraments and attended religion class every day as I had at their age. That felt comfortable, even though I still had questions on the whole religion aspect.

I had always felt that a higher power existed but could not find comfort in religion. I found comfort in prayer, and there was a period in my life where I had suffered extreme loss. I never blamed God but I had questions. I didn't understand the how or the why of it all. I felt that my losses were unfair, but I still didn't place blame anywhere. It would be years later that I would come to understand my own spirituality.

I attended church services at some point after my divorce. At the time, I felt so alone. I was hoping to find some comfort through the difficulty that I was going through. It felt so uncomfortable that I wanted to get up and leave! Again, it would be years later and personal growth work that would help me identify my faith and beliefs. I don't pray often but rather I find comfort going to the beach or just being in nature to show gratitude for the amazing world that has been created by a higher power. This brings me peace.

CANCER AND SPIRITUALITY

I know why I got cancer. I know it was all the years of striving to be perfect and holding in emotions of grief, anger, and resentment as well as the excess stress that comes with that.

I blame no one for my cancer. What I know to be true is that I didn't have the tools I needed to deal with my emotional detachment before I got cancer. I am so grateful for the personal growth work I was fortunate enough to experience prior to my diagnosis because, honestly, I don't know how I would have gotten through it. Having a more positive mindset, having faith in my medical team, using my voice to advocate for my care and allowing myself to feel all of the emotions were important factors in my healing.

I am truly grateful to my higher power for giving me exactly what I need, exactly when I need it.

There was only one time during this cancer journey that I made a deal with God. I was sitting in yet another hospital waiting room to get an MRI of my brain. I didn't know if I could survive brain cancer. The deal went like this: "God, if there is some chance you can spare me from brain cancer, I promise I will help other people going through this. Please!!!!!"

I was spared that day, and I am now paying it forward and keeping that promise.

SPIRITUALITY ROUTINE

I have two daily practices. The first is a daily practice of meditation. I realized, during my cancer battle, that a commitment to meditation fills me with peace. It allows me to be in the moment and appreciate the things around me. It is one of the first things I do to begin my day. Meditation

> I believe in faith: faith in myself, faith in my higher power, faith in the human race and faith in my higher self. If you know what you believe in, embrace it! If you are still searching, don't stop...you'll find it!

grounds me. There are a slew of meditation apps and resources you can do on your own. However, I have had the privilege of working closely with Angela Sanders, founder of Mindful Mindz, and she has helped me deepen my practice in a very powerful way. I highly recommend you look her up online.

The second is a gratitude practice. Often I do this on my way to work or at the end of the day before I go to bed. I list ten things every single day that I want to show gratitude for. Sometimes this list is written and sometimes I just say them. The number one item on my list every day is that I am so grateful for my perfect health because it is keeping me alive. Number seven is also super important to me, which states, "I am truly grateful to my higher power for giving me exactly what I need, exactly when I need it." This is how I practice my "religion," if you want to call it that.

LOOKING TO THE FUTURE

I believe that spirituality is a very personal gift. I don't think there is one way that is right for everyone and that everyone gets to decide for themselves what that looks like.

I believe in a higher power whether that is called God, Buddha, Spirit, The Universe or Infinite Intelligence. I believe in faith: faith in myself, faith in my higher power, faith in the human race and faith in my higher self. If you know what you believe in, embrace it! If you are still searching, don't stop...you'll find it!

I promised that I would pay it forward after cancer. One of the reasons that Marc and I wrote this book is because we believe there are seven aspects of life beyond cancer that require vision. Each area needs to be personalized because each of us is unique, and we are here to help you think more deeply and find what works for you.

Some people find solace in church, some may find that comfort sitting in the woods. It really doesn't matter where you are or who you are or what you pray to or honor; I believe it's all plugged into a higher power. Life happens for you; not to you. Having a vision for your spiritual life will help get you to where you want to be.

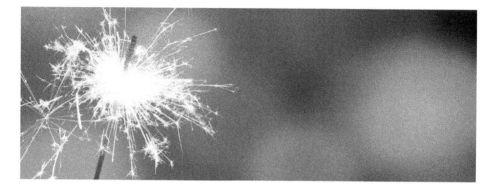

CONTRIBUTION

Only those who have learned the power of
sincere and selfless contribution experience
life's deepest joy; true fulfillment.

— *Tony Robbins*

MARC'S LIFE IN CONTRIBUTION

EARLY FAMILY LIFE

I learned about true generosity early in my life from my amazing parents. They always took care of me, my sisters, aunts, uncles, cousins and everyone else around them. They took special care of both my grandmothers. My father provided for them financially, and I have fond memories of Tuesday night fish fry at my maternal grandmother's house. No matter the holiday MY favorite chicken parmesan was on the menu at my paternal grandmother's house.

> **We realized that we had to help. I felt such a strong sense of responsibility and concern inside of me, in a way I had never felt it before.**

They were both widows early in their lives, and family was everything to us.

When someone in the family struggled, my parents helped. They took in a few of my cousins when I moved out to go to college, and I saw them make room for my aunt's family for over a year. My dad also helped two of my best friends David Heiss and Scott Fried start their very long and successful careers on the New York Stock Exchange. These experiences became the catalyst for contribution and generosity towards others for me. Philanthropy has continued to be an important part of my life.

When I started working on the New York Stock Exchange, I always contributed to those around me; whether it was sponsoring a little league team, supporting veterans or sending a school band on a trip. I was always willing to step in and I didn't think too much about it. It was just money, and to me, it was easy to give away because that's how my parents raised me. But volunteering my time and getting involved at a personal level with the community didn't happen until after the attack on the Twin Towers.

REALIZATION AFTER 9/11

September 11th, 2001 is a day that everyone remembers. I bet you know exactly where you were, right? Since I lived four blocks north of the World Trade Centers and worked three blocks south, when the towers fell and many people were watching it happen on their TV, I was right there. It was surreal. *Could this really be happening?*, I thought at the time. It all felt so personal.

We were hunkered down in the Exchange until 12:30 p.m. when we were finally told it was safe to leave. After reassuring my parents that Danielle and I were okay, we realized that we had to help. I felt such a strong sense of responsibility and concern inside of me, in a way I had never felt it before. Although many of our neighbors and friends left the city to escape the disaster, we decided to stay.

Directed to walk the long way home, we were trudging through streets covered deeply with ashes. We quickly changed our clothes and began helping people evacuate the Cosmopolitan Hotel, a shelter for homeless older people that was uninhabitable. Shortly afterward, we saw firefighters and asked what we could do to help them. They told us they were setting up a triage center in Stuyvesant High School and needed help carrying cots and medical supplies. That took us all night. During this time, we found out about volunteering through the Salvation Army and our plan the next day was to be officially connected with them and do whatever they needed us to do.

On Wednesday morning, we walked a mile to the Salvation Army. Walking there was utter chaos. There were no cabs in sight, and the subway wasn't running. We received volunteer badges and were promptly put to work helping those who needed it at Ground Zero. It's hard to explain how devastating the scene was without getting choked up about it today. There were enormous piles of rubble littering the area, rescuers everywhere trying to find survivors, and dust and debris covering everything. We saw crushed vehicles, dozens of fire engines, and people running in all directions in the hopes of rescuing one more person.

Danielle and I walked back and forth from our apartment to Ground Zero for five days. We were in the pit and rubble assisting firefighters, EMTs, and anyone who needed help. We delivered water and food to the first responders. We passed out masks, hand wipes, and medical supplies. It was something I will never forget.

As messed up as things were at that time in the United States, we saw the best of people and the best of New Yorkers. No one cared about skin color, religion, political affiliation or title. We were only focused on helping each other.

Being a volunteer support staff for those who were searching for survivors was hard work, but we wanted to help as many as we could. As messed up as things were at that time in the United States, we saw the best of people and the best of New Yorkers. No one cared about skin color, religion, political affiliation or title. We were only focused on helping each other.

Seeing that, I had a very personal revelation. I realized that contributing my time and being a part of something larger than myself had a much larger impact than just writing a check. It made me feel good to be able to help no matter how small the task. When Sunday night rolled around, I told

> **The mark had been made on my heart, and I would never forget what I felt when I was volunteering during 9/11.**

Danielle that I didn't want to go back to work. I wanted to stay and continue to volunteer and help. Although it was a noble and nice idea, I was reminded that I had eight employees and a successful business. Those employees relied on me and needed me to show up and run the business so they could support their families too. So, for the next six years, I worked at my business and Danielle and I continued to volunteer our time and support wherever we could. The mark had been made on my heart, and I would never forget what I felt when I was volunteering during 9/11.

A DOUBLE-EDGED SWORD

Ten years after this experience my cancer surfaced, and I believe it is a direct result of being exposed to the 9/11 dust cloud and living in that area of Manhattan for those six years post-9/11 that we chose to stay. Although the EPA told us that the air was clean, there's no doubt in my mind that the toxicity at Ground Zero directly caused my cancer. I have no familial history of lymphoma or any other forms of cancer.

As much as going through cancer and treatment was hell, the honest truth is, I would do it all over again. Being at Ground Zero, volunteering with the Salvation Army in the pit and helping out during a time that was a living hell for so many are experiences I'll never regret. It was more painful to see and life-changing to be a part of, than anything one could experience in their lifetime.

Comparatively, the treatment and the physical changes I had to endure throughout cancer, although difficult and painful, were nothing in light of what so many lost on that tragic day. Volunteering during 9/11 changed me so much for the better. Yes, I got sick, but I'm not bitter, I'm better. I'm still here, and I will not stop giving.

A DIFFERENT OUTLOOK

Now living in Naples, our city is repeatedly voted to be the happiest and healthiest place in the United States. It is also a very affluent area for vacationers from all over the world with some of the best beaches and shelling. But we're also right in the middle of Hurricane Alley, which means there is a season where the chances of being hit by a hurricane are likely. Most recently, our chance came in September of 2017, as we watched the news for a week when Hurricane Irma was out at sea. A few days before it was supposed to hit landfall in Miami it changed course, and within forty-eight hours came crashing through our town.

We evacuated for a few days and upon return, we saw the devastation. Our power was out for over a week, and we were bouncing around living at various friends' houses who did have power. Collier County was under a restricted water use notice; you couldn't flush the toilets as the sewage pumps were not functional and you could not drink the city water. While this was all inconvenient, it wasn't tragic...for us.

It wasn't long before I realized just twenty miles east of us was a town that was torn apart. Immokalee is largely made up of immigrants and migrant workers who have come to try and make a better life for themselves and their families. Unfortunately, the eye of the storm had passed directly through their little community. Many of their manufactured homes were destroyed, the fields they worked in were flooded and there was no way for them to bring in an income without a place to work. They were just trying to survive.

I knew what to do. Jump in and help! A group of us rallied the leaders of our community together to gather supplies. It was a flashback to 2001. For days and weeks, we collected, sorted and delivered supplies out to that small town. We managed to bring blankets, food, diapers, toiletries, pillows, fresh water, ice and a few months after the hurricane we went back and delivered some Christmas toys for the children. It felt good to be contributing again, and to see the joy on their faces was humbling.

From this experience, we have attracted a group of friends and colleagues who value contribution as highly as we do. We are always looking for ways to help our community thrive and share from our abundance. It doesn't matter if it is for hurricane survivors or others in need, we are just a group of people that want to help and contribute. Period.

WHO I AM

I am at my best when I'm in contribution. This is my highest value and knowing that my time and energy can directly impact others fires me up; it gets my blood flowing. Watching people help each other during 9/11 and Irma made me want to be my best self all the time. Contributing monetarily and volunteering my time is forever ingrained in me now.

> **Watching people help each other during 9/11 and Irma made me want to be my best self all the time. Contributing monetarily and volunteering my time is forever ingrained in me now.**

Whether you are going through cancer or giving to a cause, know that you can make a difference in someone else's life. Even if you're feeling like you're at the worst point in your life, the easiest way to take your mind off of your own pain is to contribute to others; I firmly believe that. I am encouraging you right now: be generous with your time and your energy. Realize you have life lessons and knowledge to give. Someone out there could learn from you. It's amazing what a smile can do to brighten someone else's day.

Every day I practice this. Even though cancer was one of the hardest things I have been through, I am now on the other side and I believe I have a moral obligation to help others. If I can help even one person with this book by putting my pain and hope into words, then it has been worth it!

FULL CIRCLE

It was uplifting for me to see the best of people in the worst of times. So, that's the premise of Shine Beyond Cancer. Lisa and I are taking the worst times of our lives and using it to help you. We can help, and we are willing to do so, and sometimes that's all it takes. Show up and be available.

We hope that the interviews, podcasts, and videos will help you heal and give you hope. We understand what you are going through better than most people. This is how we have chosen to contribute to the cancer community. You won't be alone through this. Allow us to help you deal with the stress of going through cancer. We are here to lift you up and get you back to being your best self. Use cancer as your catalyst to reinvent your life and include a huge dose of contribution. Your life will be better for it!

LISA'S LIFE IN CONTRIBUTION

GROWING UP CHARITABLE

My grandmother was my all-time favorite person. Not only was she my best friend, she was also an amazing role model for me. She was always involved in many charitable organizations, and I loved being right alongside her. In grade school, I was always the first to raise my hand to be involved in community projects. This cycle of contribution has followed me my whole life.

Even though there have been struggles in my life, I have always made it a priority to remain in contribution.

I remember very early in grade school when I was six or seven, my grandmother organized volunteers at the hospital. They were called Candy Stripers, and they would visit sick people in hospitals. She took great pride in her volunteering and that experience impacted me greatly. I began to see the ways that someone could lead others to do good in the world.

As I grew into a young adult, I continued to do volunteer and community work. There were always community projects that needed people to help complete the mission. I enjoyed being part of a caring group of people and helping those who needed it.

CONTINUING THE FAMILY TRADITION

When I reached adulthood and started working, I made it a priority to continue helping, whether it was participating in a community event, donating time or organizing community projects through my job. When my girls were little, I also became involved in the school system. I was always in some sort of volunteer position from coordinating fundraiser auctions to Brownie Troop leader to president of the PTO.

And of all the final words of wisdom during those three and a half months, the one that stuck with me most was "make a difference in another person's life." I loved that man!

From 1999 to 2004, I was fortunate enough to be involved on a large scale in my community by working on both local and national government campaigns. We always tried to create programs to make things better for people. Looking back, it felt good to be a part of something bigger than myself. I don't think at the time I realized that I was living in contribution. It was just something I felt good about. Even though there have been struggles in my life, I have always made it a priority to remain in contribution.

I know I inherited this trait from both my father and his mother (my beloved grandmother). It wasn't until my thirties and forties that I realized the impact my father made on the lives of people, whether he knew them or not. He wasn't on the front page of the newspaper or spearheading large community projects but rather quietly in the background changing people's lives one at a time.

In 2000, my dad and I spent many hours together while he was in hospice talking about life. He had no regrets. He had done the best he could. And of all the final words of wisdom during those three and a half months, the one that stuck with me most was "make a difference in another person's life." I loved that man!

CONTRIBUTION AND CANCER

Although I was always supporting others, I never had a specific vision for contribution; it was just something I did. If an opportunity came up, I would jump on board one hundred percent. When I went through my personal growth work, and contribution was a category that I needed to create a vision for, I sat down and said, "How can I be in contribution outside of myself for no other reason than to make a difference in someone else's life?"

> **How can I be in contribution outside of myself for no other reason than to make a difference in someone else's life?**

That was the first time I created a vision for my own role in giving time and money to others. Of all the goals I had made, that vision felt so much better than any others I have ever had for myself. I knew I wanted contribution to become an even bigger part of my life! It didn't matter to me if I was creating my own program or supporting others' efforts to contribute, I simply knew that I wanted to do even more than I was doing before.

But then I was diagnosed with cancer.

Going through treatment for cancer was a full-time job; I was a single mom with a new business, and I realized that in order to keep things together I had to be self-focused. Truth be told, I have a tendency to attract people who need attention. While I am always happy to help, it often was not reciprocated. That reality was never as clear as when it came time for me to focus on myself to get through treatment and keep everything balanced.

Some of the people who were typically on the receiving end of my generosity decided to step out of my life. I didn't have time to nurture those friendships, and somehow they didn't have time either. Despite that, I focused on keeping myself on the path I needed to be on while still being able to contribute in the ways that made sense for me then.

Contribution doesn't necessarily have to be serving meals at the homeless shelter or donating thousands of dollars; instead, it could be a word of encouragement or a compliment to someone who needs it. You don't need a dime to be able to give away something of yourself to make someone else's life a little better.

> **You don't need a dime to be able to give away something of yourself to make someone else's life a little better.**

It was in the chemo and radiation rooms that I realized I could contribute to those around me. Certainly, there were some who were feeling worse than I was, so I made a point to be a smiling face and positive influence. I became a supporter and a cheerleader in the midst of the treatment rooms and waiting areas. I would offer a word of encouragement and remind them how great it was to be alive. I look back now and see the impact I had. Even though it seemed small and insignificant at the time, I knew for sure it helped me feel better.

To this day, I have a stack of letters saved from people, who at the time didn't even know my name. They each told me that I made them feel better during their treatments. I realized then that I had made an impact! So, when I wrote them back to thank them for their kind words, I also told them that contribution comes in all shapes and sizes and I reminded them to pay it forward. Contributing to others is often more of a ripple than a tidal wave. Do what you can in small doses and you will certainly see how your actions will help others.

THE VIBRANT SIDE OF CANCER

Now that I am on the vibrant side of cancer, I believe in the principles and vision of Shine Beyond Cancer to such a degree that it is all I can do to stop myself from jumping out of my skin. This vision to be a support system for those going through cancer and a vehicle to teach people to change their mindset and soar through treatment and beyond is now my life's mission. Marc and I want to use our experience to shine the light of hope and healing, and to spread inspiration and knowledge throughout the cancer community.

Your vision doesn't have to be that big; in fact, it took us many years of serving in other capacities before this project became a reality. So we encourage you to start small and start today. There is always something you can do. There are support groups you can join to become a light in the room.

The American Cancer Society always needs mentors; there are other cancer organizations that need your time and expertise, and there are many other ways that you can contribute. It doesn't cost you anything but your energy. Just being there for someone who needs it can make a huge impact. And it doesn't necessarily have to be centered around cancer. There are projects and organizations that need help. Whether it's donating supplies to those in need, serving a meal, cleaning up a city park or volunteering at your child's school, your contribution matters! I believe it is what makes the world go 'round.

CHARITY PROJECTS

Although I do contribute to many cancer organizations, much of what I do has nothing to do with cancer. There are needs everywhere. In 2017, when southwest Florida was hit by Hurricane Irma, I was there and I had the opportunity to get involved in a big way.

My house and business were fine structurally, although we were without power for weeks. I didn't want to focus on what I didn't have; instead, I wanted to help those who had lost far more than their electricity.

Marc, Danielle and I, together with our dear friend Michael Schaeffer, gathered people in our community to help a small town who had nothing. Their jobs were gone because they worked in the agricultural fields, so they didn't have money to buy food or supplies. Entire families were affected. So, we asked our community to help and we took goods and services to people who so desperately needed them at that time.

I'm happy to report that we bypassed every other organization out there and took what these people needed directly to them. We collected over $400,000 worth of goods. We sorted them in a raw space donated to us by our local mall and transported them with donated vehicles. One hundred percent of the money that was donated went directly to the people affected.

There were whole families living in temporary housing with no blankets or pillows, so we managed to raise and donate 700 of these items to the schoolchildren. Not long after the hurricane, it was Christmas and we collected 3,200 gifts to donate to the kids in the area that had been devastated by Hurricane Irma. It always seems like, after a disaster strikes an area, organizations and people come in to help for a little while but just as quickly they disappear. We decided we weren't going anywhere until either our resources ran out or there was no longer a need. We kept going until the community was well on its way to restoration.

FINAL THOUGHTS ABOUT CONTRIBUTION

Contribution doesn't have to mean raising $400,000 for hurricane victims. It can be words of encouragement or a simple smile in a room of scared and nervous people. It's the exact same thing. No matter how you contribute, know that YOU have a chance to make a difference in another person's life.

From a Facebook post on my page, May 9, 2014, one year after learning I was about to get on the roller coaster ride called Cancer.

"A year ago today I stood in a dimly lit radiology room at NCH. After an emergency mammogram and ultrasound, a radiologist said to me, "I cannot rule out cancer. You need to see a breast surgeon." In shock, I said, "How do I do that?" I never heard the answer if he gave one.

I have had people say to me today, "what a difference a year makes."

I remember a year ago thinking "what a difference a day makes."

And today I say, "what difference can I make?"

Life is all about perception."

I believe that contribution is the best way to get out of your own way. It's tempting when you're going through cancer to wallow in self-pity and see others as more fortunate. Don't get stuck in that trap. Helping others will promote your own healing. It brings good into your life, and the universe will give it back tenfold. I truly believe that receiving good things in our life is the universe's way of telling you that you are doing a good job. That is a great feeling, just being able and willing to help people. So I encourage you to get out there and make a difference.

No matter how you contribute, know that YOU have a chance to make a difference in another person's life.

CONCLUSION

IT'S TIME TO SHINE

Cancer is a profound, amazing, exhausting, emotional and enlightening journey. No matter where you are on this ride, we know you have the desire to shine beyond, just like we have. Hopefully, you have been inspired to take a look at each area of your life and see where you can dig a little deeper, or create a more authentic vision and perhaps write about your experience.

Our wish for you is that you will be able to make sense of this experience and use it to catapult your life beyond your wildest dreams. We will be here as an ongoing source for you to make that happen. Please visit our website www.shinebeyondcancer.com/toolbox, like our Facebook Page at Shine Beyond Cancer or follow us on Instagram to be continually supported and inspired.

We will be releasing a companion workbook to *Shine Beyond Cancer* in July 2019. You can sign up to receive updates and information by sending an email to info@shinebeyondcancer.com. In the subject line type **Sign Me Up To Shine.**

To your continued health, well-being and joy,
Keep Shining,
Lisa and Marc

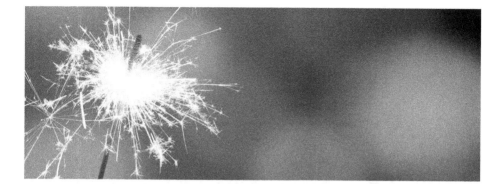

PHOTO BOOK

Lisa shining beyond cancer with a big vision.

Marc as the proud father of the bride, Samantha, October 28, 2017.

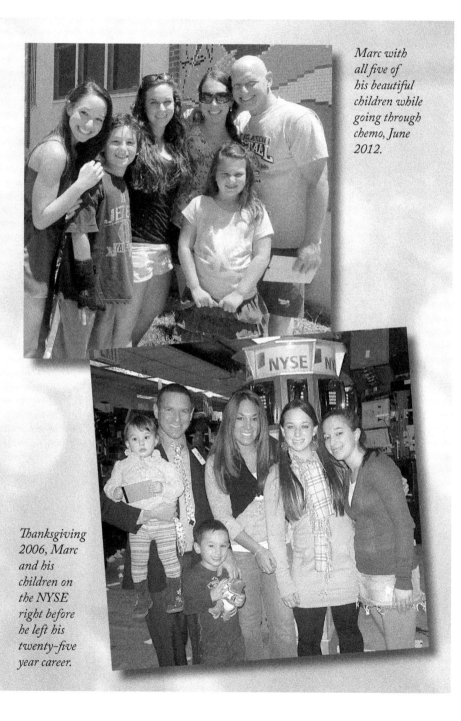

Marc with all five of his beautiful children while going through chemo, June 2012.

Thanksgiving 2006, Marc and his children on the NYSE right before he left his twenty-five year career.

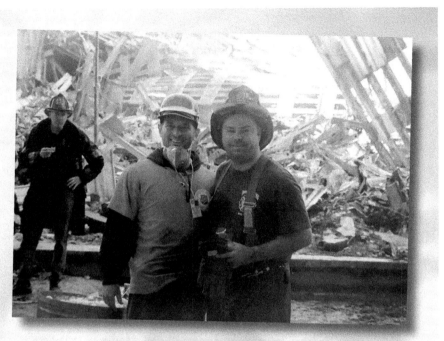

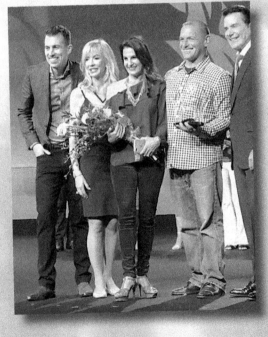

September 2001 – days after the attack on the Twin Towers, while volunteering Marc runs into a friend from the old neighborhood, Firefighter Jimmy (Roast Beef).

Marc and Danielle being recognized as Isagenix Millionaires #253, January 2018.

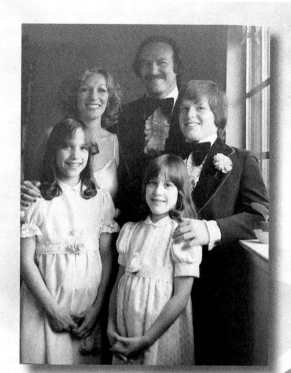

Marc's Bar Mitzvah 1976.

Danielle, Lisa and Marc jetting home from the Kentucky Derby 2018.

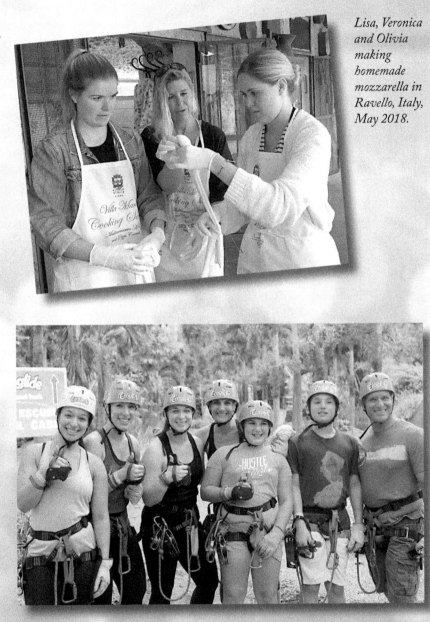

Lisa, Veronica and Olivia making homemade mozzarella in Ravello, Italy, May 2018.

Slugh family vacation, Costa Rica, 2016.

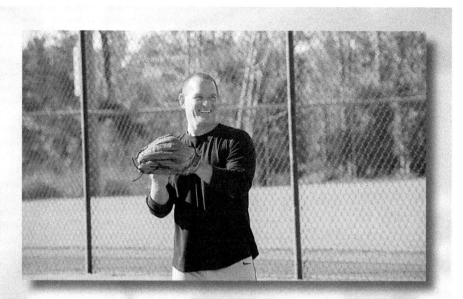

Marc enjoying his time on the softball field.

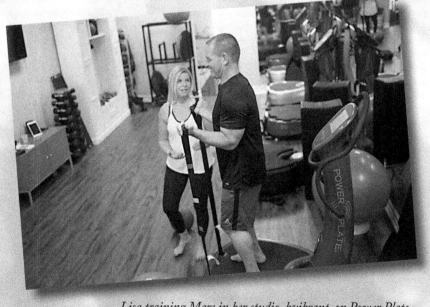

Lisa training Marc in her studio, bvibrant, on Power Plate.

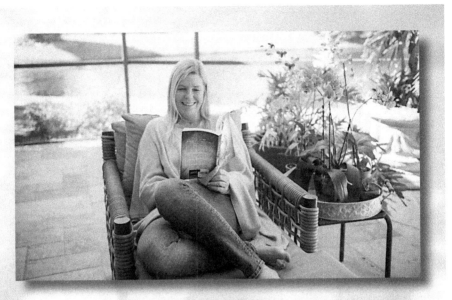

Lisa enjoying one of her favorite books, The Magic.

*Marc and Lisa post Hurricane Irma
unloading supplies, September 2017.*

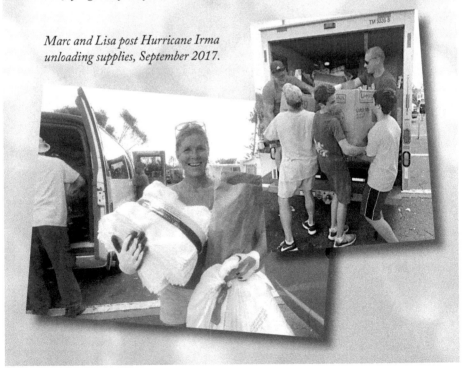

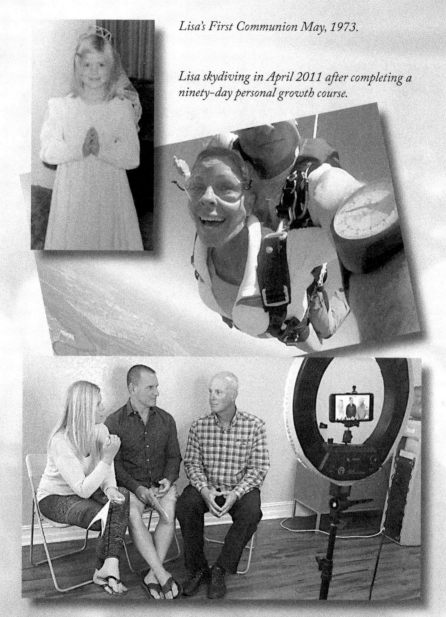

Lisa's First Communion May, 1973.

Lisa skydiving in April 2011 after completing a ninety-day personal growth course.

Lisa and Marc interviewing Dr. Frank on the Shine Beyond Cancer video series.

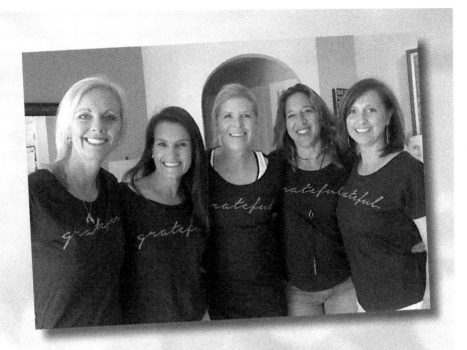

Lisa and her Power Hour women's group.

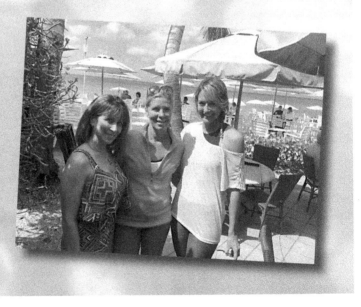

Lisa, Molly and Louise, Turtle Club, Naples, FL.

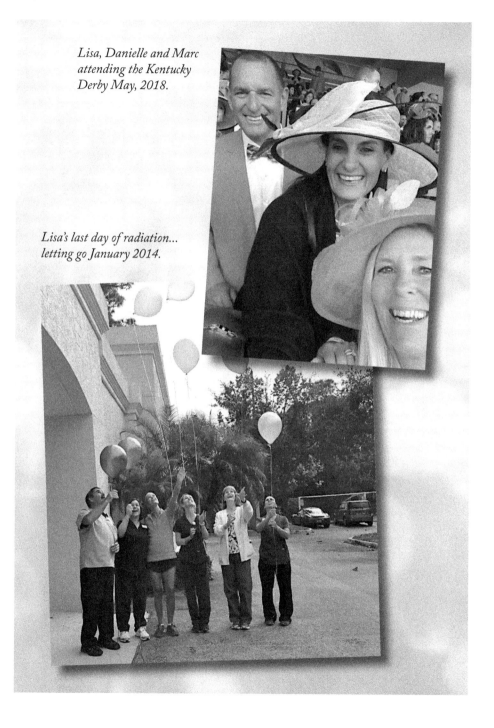

Lisa, Danielle and Marc attending the Kentucky Derby May, 2018.

Lisa's last day of radiation... letting go January 2014.

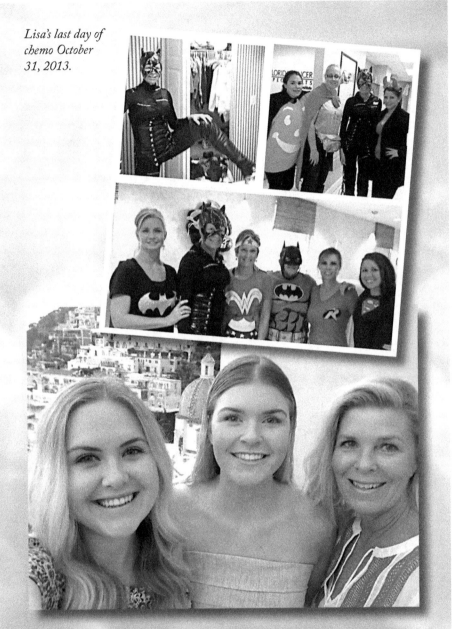

Lisa's last day of chemo October 31, 2013.

Lisa and her daughters in Positano, Italy May 2018.

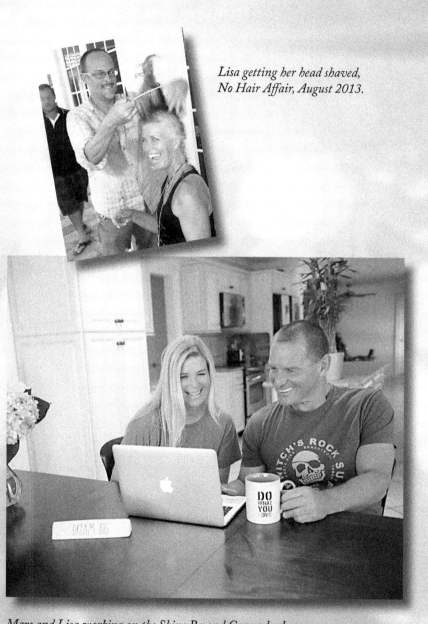

Lisa getting her head shaved, No Hair Affair, August 2013.

Marc and Lisa working on the Shine Beyond Cancer book.

MARC'S GRATITUDE

First off, thank you so much to my parents, Norm and Judy. You have taught me a 'slew' of things in my life, none more important than the understanding of generosity, unconditional love and the importance of family.

To my sisters, Marcy and Melissa, who both volunteered, no questions asked, to be my stem cell donors. Thank you for being the leaders of our generation of SHEEP. You two are amazing people.

To my in-laws, Louis and Susan, thank you for your unwavering support in so many ways when we needed it most. You will hold a special place in my heart forever.

To all the amazing people who touched my life through the Momentum/ Synergy coaching programs in NYC. The sense of community and love has touched me more than you know. Special shout out to Peter, Angel and my long lost sister and mentor, Fran Peltz.

When this book looked like a big mess and required more than Lisa and I to make this happen, the talented April O'Leary of O'Leary Publishing stepped in and made this book a reality. I am forever grateful for her help.

You know when you meet someone and right away, you know why? Well, that's what happened when I met my partner Lisa Dimond. You're an integral part of my life right now, and I thank you for always challenging me, always confiding in me and just being AMAZING.

To my five awesome, intelligent, remarkable children, Samantha, DJ, Brittany, Nick, and Sarah. You are my inspiration, my WHY, my reason I kicked cancer's ass.

To my wife, Danielle. Wow. What can I say? How do I ever express my gratitude? You're my love, my confidant, my best friend. You always see the best in me and are always right there if I go off track. You keep me focused on what is important. Your energy and smile are contagious. You make my life more vibrant, adventurous and fun beyond my wildest dreams. I adore you and love you more than you will ever know.

LISA'S GRATITUDE

I can't help but think of a Kenny Chesney song as I begin to write this: *I Didn't Get Here Alone.* And I certainly couldn't have done it on my own.

Veronica and Olivia, you are my heart, my joy and the purest inspiration in my life. You were my reason for the relentless fight. I often say I've made a lot of mistakes but there are two things I got right. I am blessed and honored to be your mother, and I love you to the moon and back.

I was surrounded by so much love and support but Louise Messina, you were the glue that held everything together by constantly rearranging your schedule to be at doctor appointments, tests, surgeries and treatments with me. You provided nurturing support for my girls, and even if you didn't always agree with my decisions, you let me do this "my way." I will be forever grateful and I love you with all my heart.

And when I just wanted to feel "normal," Molly Coates, you were always there with just the right adventure or the calming words I needed to hear. Thank you for encouraging me to celebrate all the victories (even the small ones) and for loving me just the way I am. Who says you can't meet a stranger on the beach and become best friends? Love you so much!

Thank you, Tina Crumpacker, Jaime, and Carlos for all of the gifts, blessings, and lessons that you poured into The Journey – Advanced Living Principles – Leadership.

To Dr. Alan Brown, Dr. Chaundre Cross and the rest of my amazing medical team, thank you! I wasn't always the easiest patient to deal with, but I appreciate every ounce of effort you put into my care.

Thank you, Vandy Beach crew and the No Hair Affair gang. You all know who you are. I will forever be touched by your unconditional love and support!

Gator, I will never forget that day on the park bench at the beach! Our souls were definitely meant to meet. Keep shining, my friend! I love you!

I need to acknowledge my clients, past and present. Thank you for your trust and allowing me to be part of your health and wellness journey. I am so grateful that my experience allows me to feel a deeper compassion for your well-being.

Shifra Becker, thank you for making me get on that BEMER! My life was changed forever! I love you, mama!!!

Lisa Moore and Leslie Fox, I am so grateful for all of your love and support and for helping me figure out how I could first, afford a BEMER and second, how to change other lives eight minutes at a time.

If you think cancer is difficult, try writing a book about it. Thank you, April O'Leary and the entire team at O'Leary Publishing for having a process to make this project easier and for believing in our vision! You guys rock!

Danielle Russo-Slugh, I am so grateful for your love and support; for your amazing nutrition coaching; for reminding me to "dream big;" and for constantly connecting and promoting! You are the best "D-Rock" on the planet! And thank you for sharing your husband as we wrote this book and launched Shine Beyond Cancer.

And lastly but certainly not least, Marc Slugh, when I think of all the things that the Universe had to line up for you and I to write this book, I'm overwhelmed with emotion. The depth of my respect, love, and gratitude for you is immeasurable. Sometimes you just know things were meant to be. Looking forward to our next chapter. Let's change some lives! Shine on and much love, my friend!

CONTACT US

We're thrilled you took the time to read *Shine Beyond Cancer*. We are always looking to feature cancer survivors with inspiring stories on our podcast and video series. If you, or someone you know, would be a great guest please fill out the contact form at www.shinebeyondcancer.com/toolbox.

O'Leary Publishing provides concierge book publishing services for brands, professionals, and entrepreneurs. We bring you from idea to print effortlessly through a proven system that is especially effective for non-writers and those who would prefer to leave the writing to an expert. For more about our services visit www.olearypublishing.com.

The O'Leary Publishing Team

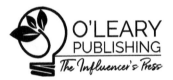

CPSIA information can be obtained
at www.ICGtesting.com
Printed in the USA
LVHW032144130219
607448LV00015B/37/P